GINÁSTICA NATURAL

THE ULTIMATE BODY WEIGHT TRAINING FOR PERFORMANCE AND QUALITY OF LIFE

ALVARO ROMANO

ISBN 13: 978-0692844014
ISBN 10: 0692844015

Photos and Ilustration – Juilo Fonyat,

Inside photos Kid Peligro, Flavio Scorsato, Raphael Gandara and private archives of the author

Cover Design – Renata Romano

Translation from Portuguese

GINÁSTICA NATURAL

Table of Contents

Chapter 7

Chapter 8

Chapter 9

Chapter 10

Chapter 11

Chapter 12

Chapter 13

Chapter 14

Chapter 15

Chapter 16

Chapter 17

Chapter 18

Chapter 19

Dedication

In memory of my father, Alvaro Romano, for his example of love and dedication to his family.

To my mother Marlene, for her unconditional love for me and my children.

To my son Raphael and my daughter Renata, for always serving as a source of inspiration, with their love and affection and for their ongoing support.

Acknowledgements

To my daughter Renata Romano for her contribution to *Ginastica Natural*, Paulo Guillobel author of *Mastering the 21 Immutable Principles of Brazilian Jiu Jitsu* for encouraging me to write this book; all the students, athletes and professors who believed in me and served as the main inspiration for me to develop my work in the area of Physical Education and Health, and the Photographer Julio Fonyat, Monika Zeldini, Gracie Family, Kid Peligro, Fabio Santos, Raphael Gandara, Dr. Darcymires, Rego Barros (in memoriam), Professor Roberto Pavel, Professor Orlando Cani, Dr Angelo Vargas.

To Rolls Gracie (in memoriam) who, through jiu-jitsu, contributed toward my training as an athlete and Professor.

Recognition

My son Raphael Romano, who has practiced *Ginastica Natural* since he was five years old. By joining the world of Physical Education, he became a crucial player in the evolution of the method through his studies in the areas of training, quality of life and health, and his certification courses for instructor training. Through his work, he has helped disseminate *Ginastica Natural* and promoted the quality of life and health for those who practice it around the world.

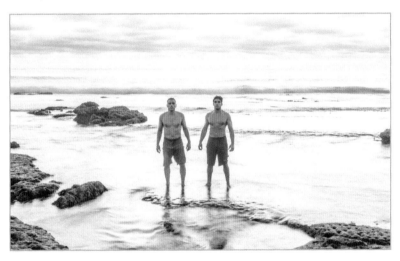

Alvaro Romano and Raphael Romano

PREFACE

It is a pleasure and honor unlike any other to write the preface for a work as special as this one here, now being presented to the academic and scientific communities. Nevertheless, this is not an easy task, considering the magnitude of the book's scope and also Professor Alvaro Romano's importance in the area of physical activities, not only within the Brazilian context, but also on an international level.

For some time now, I have had the privilege of working closely with the author professionally, and we have also shared the joy of embarking on our academic-university development together. Needless to say, I am a big admirer of Professor Alvaro Romano and was lucky enough to serve as witness and apprentice to his exceptional contributions to the episteme of Physical Education within the global context. If we delve back in history to 19th century Herbert, you find an empirical researcher concerned with the customary deterioration of the human race, so hooked on "modern" lifestyles that greatly limit our transcendent capacities, as asserted by Manuel Sergio in his "Epistemology of Human Motricity." Along these same lines, Professor Alvaro Romano did not only structure the foundations of the *Ginastica Natural* method, but also faithfully assumed the responsibility of systemizing it, leading to its insertion into the areas of health, sports and lifestyle. This work, therefore, addresses topics like health, quality of life, nature and diet. It also covers the practice of sports and other aspects of our planetary existence.

Last but not least, it is important to add that the book I have had the honor of prefacing deserves substantial recognition in our globalized society.

Finally, I would like to reiterate my tribute to the author, and not only because we share an idealism based on the universe of martial arts and sports. We are very proud indeed of our university degrees, but, most importantly, it is his idealism and commitment to building knowledge and preserving human life that I find so impressive.

///

Angelo Vargas / Member of the Federal Physical Education Board / Brazil
Post-Doctorate in Sports Sciences and Post-Doctorate in Sociology / Professor at the Federal University of Rio de Janeiro and Estácio de Sa University

PRESENTATION

CONFEF

Federal Council of Physical Education / Brazil

Mr. Alvaro Robin Romano Junior, Professional of Physical Education, registered at the Regional Council of Physical Education of the first Region, under the n.CREF 000712-G/RJ is Mentor, Diffuser and Adviser of the Ginastica Natural method.

THE FEDERAL COUNCIL OF PHYSICAL EDUCATION – CONFEF and the REGIONAL COUNCILS OF PHYSICAL EDUCATION – CREFs, created by the Federal law n.9696 dated September 1,1998, are the entities empowered by the Union to regulate, advise, discipline, and inspect the practice of the activities inherent to Physical Education Professionals and to legal entities, which basic purpose consists in rendering services to the areas of physical, sporting, and similar activities, with administrative, financial, and patrimony autonomy, acting as the CONFEF/CREFs system.

The Federal Council of Physical Education – CONFEF is the highest deliberative, normative, judging and executive stage of the national system that, in its expression and complexity, gathers representations of all professional segments of the Physical Education area.

The CONFEF/CREFs system shall develop programs on continuing education, making possible to the Physical Education Professionals to update their knowledge, and it states that the Professional ALVARO ROMANO is one of the professionals who are qualified for this purpose, considering his well know skill and national and international acknowledgement regarding the quality of life and wellbeing.

//

Jorge Steinhilber
President Federal Council Of Physical Education –
Cref-000002-G/Rj

INTRODUCTION

Currently, there are a growing number of exercise modalities practiced in fitness centers around the world. Most are outdated, and end up needing to be reinvented. By adding a new appearance in standards, equipment, music, how the exercise is approached or by giving it a new nickname, the modalities are proliferated as activities and/or modern methods of physical conditioning.

Most of the media created for exercise are born of the creativity of the instructors. Their practical experiences and organized sequences of movements have, over time, been validated by scientists using academic experiments. Without a doubt, this has assisted in the declaration of these methods. Exercise is an efficient means for the improvement of physical fitness, as it also improves the quality of life of its practitioners.

The man moves his body, according to his empirical history, and explained by anthropology, has changed through the ages. At the beginning, man used rudimentary forms of movements. After a few centuries, form was improved. Some historians believed that history relates to the intellectual development of mankind, which has been changing in every manner; even in the way humankind sees the world. In terms of body movement, not much has changed. In other words, man has always moved very naturally. Currently, modernization has led many in our culture to adopt a sedentary lifestyle resulting in serious problems for this generation in pathological diseases not yet fully understood by current medicine.

In recent times, the practice of physical exercises has become a rule in society. Technology helped the practice to gain notoriety. Several practical methods of exercises in which technology plays a role, were formatted with contradictory movements to natural movements, thus, ignoring the nature of the human body, and consequently, the natural essence of human movement.

In this work, Prof. Alvaro Romano, a scholar with decades of experience in the area of physiology/kinesiology, relates how some recently created methods degrade natural movement. He tries to rescue organic movements of human beings aggregated with movements of other animal species which form ginastica natural. Indeed natural, even in name, because the essential movements are performed in an instinctive way; practiced anywhere without equipment and with a peculiar creativity to it.

This work comes at an important moment in the evolution of methods of body exercises and aims at the improvement of the physical condition of humanity. Consequently, these activities improve the quality of life of its practitioners. We need to change the stereotypes involving exercise. Society perpetrates workouts as more to do with technological devices. These mechanisms restrict the natural physical capabilities that are necessary to human life.

I have the honor to introduce this researched data to those professionals in the area of sports, fitness and wellness. It is produced by Prof. Alvaro Romano and is indispensable; it presents us with his vast experience and knowledge. You will be inspired to reflect on the methods of body exercises and existing technology in today's market.

Antonio Carlos Gomes, PhD
Brazilian Coaching Academy (ABT)
Brazilian Olympic Institute (IOB)

ABOUT THE AUTHOR

Alvaro Romano was born in 1956, in the city of Rio de Janeiro, Brazil. He earned a B.A. in Physical Education at Gama Filho University (Brazil) and a graduate degree from Estacio de Sá University (Brazil) in Physical Education and Recreation. He is a Jiu-Jitsu 6th Degree Black Belt, Judo Brown Belt, triathlete, open water swimmer and soccer player. He has surfed since 1970 and was one of the pioneers in the physical training work for surfing and jiu-jitsu athletes in Brazil. He has given lectures, courses and workshops about *Ginastica Natural*, physical fitness, functional training, quality of life, health and well-being in several countries, including: Brazil, Chile, Argentina, Peru, Ecuador, Mexico, United States, Canada, Italy, Sweden, Switzerland, Norway, Austria, Germany, Hungary, France, Russia, Spain, Portugal, England, Scotland, Poland, Arab Emirates, Indonesia, China, Japan, Singapore, South Korea and Saint Martin. Alvaro is the author of a collection of videos on *Ginastica Natural*, the book entitled *"Ginastica Natural"* and one of the authors of "An Anthology on Physical Activities." He has given classes for the Physical Education and Physical Therapy courses at Estácio de Sá University (Rio de Janeiro). He also took part as physical trainer during events around the globe featuring some of the main jiu-jitsu, MMA and surfing athletes. He has resided in the United States since 2007 and gave a seminar about his *Ginastica Natural* method for FBI, DEA and SWATT agents and has representatives of his method in 29 different countries through certification courses.

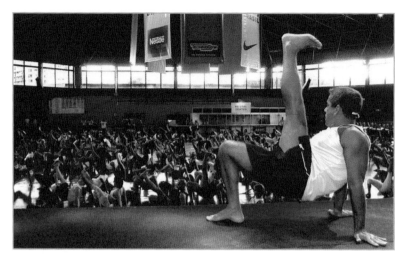

GINASTICA NATURAL WORSHOP IN BRAZIL

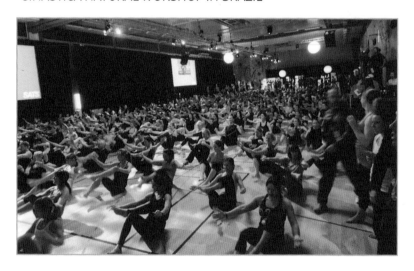

GINASTICA NATURAL WORKSHOP IN SWEDEN

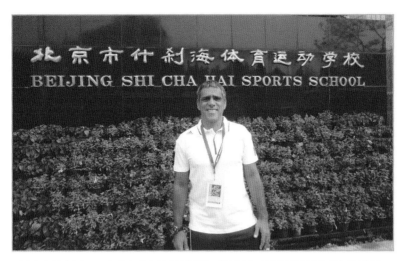

PROFESSOR ALVARO ROMANO TEACHING WORKSHOP IN CHINA

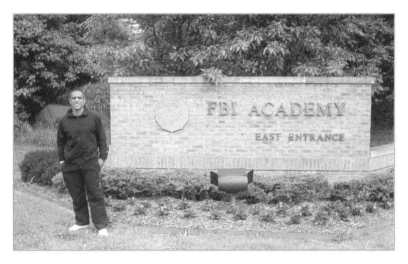

*PROFESSOR ALVARO ROMANO TEACHING SEMINAR
IN FBI ACADEMY, USA*

CHAPTER 1

A REFLECTION ON HEALTH AND QUALITY OF LIFE

I have been trying to write a book for many years now, but constant travels, personal life changes, and primarily, events and work to improve the method I developed had always led me to believe that work would never be ready. After all, I constantly want to update it. This is normal, since as time passes, everything evolves in all areas. However, in the areas of human movement, this change has occurred at an impressive speed. It can be said that many of these new methods, such as training using the body's own weight, breathing techniques, functional training, outdoor activities in contact with nature and radical sports were already practiced and were the concept behind many methods in the past that have regained popularity today. Since 1977, when I started my university studies in Physical Education, I began to study and research several types of training and activities to find the path I would follow as a Physical Education professional. My idea has always been to develop a method with concepts and foundations that come from the activities I practiced, and which could offer practitioners physical conditioning, well-being, health and quality of life. Furthermore, I sought a method that could offer the necessary understanding of how physical activity can improve our life. Routine and the consequent lack of motivation increasingly thwart people from practicing physical activity. The majority of the population understands that there is no magic formula for losing weight or having a body with toned muscles from one day to the next. First off, we need to understand that both during performance training as well as the regular practice of physical activities, we need to respect our limits. One's physical appearance is the consequence of several different factors, and the quest for good health, well-being and physical fitness has to be something constant and daily. The purpose of physical activity is not just to build muscles, but also to improve spiritual and mental health.

Movement is present in all phases of our life, from our time in-utero, when we extend and retract our arms and legs, similarly to the movement used to swim. After birth, we drag ourselves, crawl, find our balance and finally walk, all part of the evolution of our motor movements. Each one of these phases is important, and with each phase, we develop muscle groups that will be crucial for the next phase. Therefore, it is important to continue working with this "machinery," since a body that does not move does not renew its energy. The muscles wither and, over the course of a lifetime, difficulties completing simple tasks can become an obstacle for quality of life. The convenience of modern life when it comes to our routine tasks has made us sedentary.

The movements of animals have influenced martial arts and many of those movements that we practice in modern day were done spontaneously and occasionally by primitive man. These include activities like walking along rough terrain, crawling to hide in vegetation or between trees, climbing trees to collect fruit, jumping from great heights and maneuvering across abysses and through obstacles, lifting and hauling rocks and trunks, running quickly or for long periods after prey or to escape storms or the enemy, using the hand and fist to punch or complete certain tasks, body-to-body combat with men and animals, swimming in rivers and lakes and diving to catch fish.

Because human beings are biopsychosocial animals, graced with autonomy and intelligence, they must be dealt with in their entirety, actively interacting with nature. Human health can only be envisaged within this three-part dimension. However, I have included a few concepts here that I use and seek to pass on to my students, both amateurs who practice physical activity and athletes alike, so they can improve their health, quality of life and performance.

ADEQUATE NUTRITION

Many people use the word "diet," but I prefer the term "adequate nutrition" to perhaps facilitate understanding. It is important for people to enjoy what they eat, although not all that tastes good is healthy. It is all a question of moderation and good sense. Athletes burn more calories, so their case is different than a person who simply walks each day. It is important to understand the importance of balancing what you expend in energy with what you will consume, without being too radical. We all know the healthy foods, this is not new to anyone, but we may at times eat pasta or meat, with such options based on each person's taste. I have not eaten red meat since the 1990s, but this is my personal choice. Changing eating habits can be hard for many, and may be done slowly and gradually, remembering always that nutrition is the foundation for everything – it is what will control our health.

REST

Rest is crucial and an important factor for ensuring everyone's health and quality of life. In modern day, we spend several hours at the computer and sleep little. It is through rest that we recover our energy and well-being. Nevertheless, many people do not respect this and they overdo it, not allowing themselves to rest after a day of work or physical activity. It is easy to detect when we need to rest: fatigue, irritability and lack of concentration are but a few of the many symptoms detected.

RECREATION

Thinking that health and quality of life are achieved only when we are exercising is a big mistake. If this were the case, we would not find so many people in shape and with well-tone tummies, yet seemingly always in a bad mood, not enjoying life and with precarious health. It is indeed possible for people with toned bodies to be unhealthy, and therefore, we also need the social side, our family, friends, leisure time, the time we just sit back and relax, dinners with good conversation or simply a time to relax.

POSITIVE MENTAL ATTITUDES

There are thoughts that will attract both good and bad things. If you head out to your activity or daily training with a positive outlook, even if you feel tired, this can make a big difference. Remember that physical activity is an excellent way to combat fatigue, discouragement or many other diseases of an emotional nature. We all know that sensation of feeling much better after practicing some exercise. So, don't allow depression to take over. Always remember the "after-feeling," and use this to adopt a positive attitude for your entire day – both at work and when with your family.

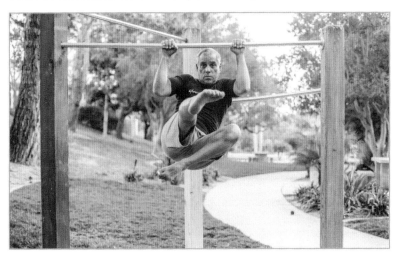

Professor Alvaro Romano, 60 years old, training in San Diego, CA

CHAPTER 2

THE INFLUENCE OF SPORTS LIKE SURFING AND JIU-JITSU

I began to train for jiu-jitsu in 1976 with the legendary Rolls Gracie the year after I enrolled at the university to study Physical Education. During this time, I began studying and applying the specific training during the jiu-jitsu competitions and my free surfing, which was important for my later work with the main Brazilian athletes in these sports.

At this time, we did not have access to information like we do today, and there was plenty of experimentation that was later adapted with athletes from the two sports. In the end, this generated an extremely interesting quantitative study to develop the techniques used in my method.

During the 1970s, the majority of surfing and jiu-jitsu athletes practiced the sport itself as a means to physical fitness, together with outdoor exercises like running and parallel bars. Many used one sport to help with the physical preparation of another, several jiu-jitsu athletes used surfing as a tool to help them with their performance and vice-versa, and hang-gliders also used jiu-jitsu as an important element in their physical preparation.

Until I was 13, I lived in a suburb of Rio de Janeiro. I did not have access to athletic clubs or any other place that offered martial arts or sports. I was involved with those activities every other suburban kid did – outdoor exercises through many different games, street soccer and others. It was when I moved to the city's Southern Zone, the neighborhood of Ipanema close to the famous surfing point Arpoador Beach, that I first came into contact with sports like surfing and capoeira.

The first contact I had with capoeira was through a friend. I went to practice in a *favela* (slum) close to my home, since there were no gyms nearby with this activity. We walked up the hill into the *favela* to learn with the Master who lived there. I was 14 years old at the time. There were also groups that met almost daily at Arpoador Beach to practice capoeira. This is an activity that is very physically demanding, developing several different motor skills and offering practitioners excellent fitness training.

I became familiar with jiu-jitsu first through Relson Gracie, who was the first Gracie to surf and the one responsible for integrating surfing with jiu-jitsu in Rio de Janeiro. Relson's nickname was "Champion" and he lived near Arpoador like me and was at the beach surfing almost every day. The surfers knew Gracie, but training was still not part of the routine. I first came into contact with Master Rolls Gracie when surfer Renan Pitangui, who had contact with Rolls, recommended a house for him to stay at in Peru during one surfing season in 1976. During this period, I also happened to be there, and while I was walking along a street in Punta Hermosa, the surfing city that is located about two hours from Lima, I met a friend who was with Rolls. We stopped to talk for a while, discussed Relson, and by coincidence, he said he was staying at the same house I was. After that, we spent a month together surfing and living in the same house.

Rolls Gracie was a natural leader and had impressive charisma. We became friends and this surfing season ended up changing the course of my life.

The first contact I had with the "Gracie Diet," created by his father Carlos Gracie, was when he invited me to go to the small city supermarket. We bought lots of fruit and cheese, and afterward, we went to a local restaurant and he asked for plates and utensils and began to teach me about the fruit and food combos and the importance of a diet not only for athletes' health, but also for their lifestyle. During that time, even though surfers already had a healthy notion of life, even because of the philosophy surrounding the sport, we did not yet have sufficient guidance or access to much information.

During this month that we lived in the same house together with two other friends, Fabio Santos and Gilberto Lessa, who both also ended up earning a degree in Physical Education and training for jiu-jitsu, he explained to us how this sport was efficient and could change people's lives, promote unity, and of course, teaching us how, in practice, to maneuver through the misunderstandings that were often inevitable.

Rolls Gracie was very calm, he respected everyone, but what most called our attention was his desire for challenge. We surfed in Peru for some time. Since I had been there in 1972, I had found out about the most dangerous spots with the rocks. Even though his technique wasn't great, Rolls surfed all types of waves and even in all the dangerous places. Often times, the locals became furious with him, since he always nabbed the best surfing points. While out there on the water, we tried to explain to the locals who he was so they would not lose control and show attitude. This happened with one, who got really fired up and starting complaining and threatening him. I explained that he could knock a guy out easily, and without understanding what I was talking about, the guy somehow got the point and continued on his way.

There are so many stories from this trip, but for me and my friends who were there, the most important one was when we said goodbye to him and he told us:

When you get back to Brazil, go straight to my gym in Copacabana and I'll train you so you can learn more about Gracie jiu-jitsu.

CHAPTER 3

STARTING OUT IN JIU-JITSU AND THE INITIAL TRAINING

At the end of 1976 and start of 1977, I went to the famous Gracie Gym in Copacabana with my friend Fábio Santos for our first training class, at the same time that I was enrolling at Gama Filho University in Rio de Janeiro to study Physical Education.

Gracie shared the gym with Master Carlson Gracie and offered classes on Mondays, Wednesdays and Fridays, and both already had a team with some of the best fighters in the city. It was an incredible learning experience to train and interact with these athletes.

My first day was both intense and interesting, since at the time, the tactic to prove the efficiency of jiu-jitsu was to have a more advanced student show the beginner student through demonstrations. However, this advanced student would always be much "weaker" and younger. After seeing this training tactic, we had no doubts about the efficiency of this art.

The Physical Education course and training applied during my own preparation at the start were the perfect combination of practice and theory when it came to the physical preparation for fights, the importance of specific training, biomechanics and physiology studies, with sufficient data to then apply to the preparation of other athletes of different sports types.

One example from this period were the warm-ups by running around a small room, star jumps, push-ups or running with a friend on our backs, which over time was replaced with stretching and exercises using our own body weight.

I had practice as my point of departure for understanding and developing these exercises and also a concept of physical preparation, since beyond jiu-jitsu, the techniques from the judo I practiced at the university originated in Japan. Many of these had new methods for warm-ups, with exercises that used one's own body weight and which were specific for fighting. I also played soccer in the sand, went surfing and did strength training on the parallel bars located at the ends of the beach, and this experience and the results from this training method were important for my professional life.

Training for jiu-jitsu at this time meant being close to all members of the Gracie family. At the gym where I trained, Carlos Gracie Júnior helped with the classes, and all of the brothers and cousins also took part in this training, often times with supervision from Master Hélio and Master Carlos Gracie. Training for jiu-jitsu with everyone together was undoubtedly a privilege and unique opportunity.

Rolls Gracie had an older team and one that was still training, and it was this new team that represented him until his death in 1982.

We began to use stretching during the warm-ups based on a book by an American author that became available in Brazil. We took the book to the tatami mat and we stretched out based on the instructions found in its pages. That was when the warm-ups started to change, since most of the time, we were the ones who led them because we were studying Physical Education.

Rolls Gracie constantly strove for excellence while training in the art, and he understood the importance of physical preparation. When the first exercise equipment began to arrive, small gyms started popping up and we began to do this type of training together. We also went on runs every Monday morning, up a hill through a forested area of Rio de Janeiro.

For a better understanding for those who practice jiu-jitsu, Gracie was the one who created that famous interval training that begins by facing a kneeling partner that many gyms adopt. When there was some competition scheduled, the students wanted to train more often and he organized these training sessions on Saturday evenings. Because this was a leisure or family day for many, the idea was to do an intense, but short training session, lasting a maximum of 40 minutes. This training session included a quick warm-up, and then we stood face-to-face with a partner. After his signal, the training began and each round lasted 10 minutes on average. In the end, the athletes changed positions with another partner and the new round started immediately with a very short period of rest.

Rolls Gracie transformed the lives of an entire generation in Rio de Janeiro. He left this world in 1982 after a hang-gliding accident, but his legacy and his example lived on among all students and friends.

I received my brown belt from Master Carlos Gracie Júnior one week after the death of Gracie, who had trained me. When the gym moved to Barra da Tijuca, a different neighborhood of

Rio de Janeiro, I started training with Master Rickson Gracie, when I earned my black belt.

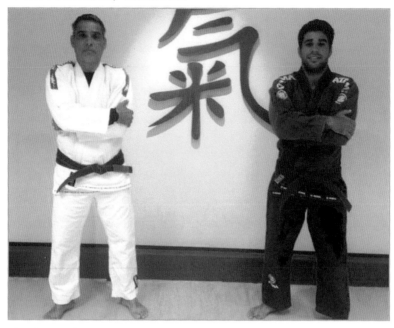

Professor Alvaro Romano and Raphael Romano

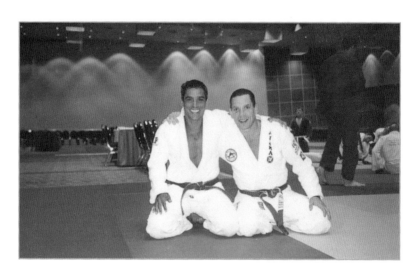

Alvaro Romano and Master Relson Gracie after training session

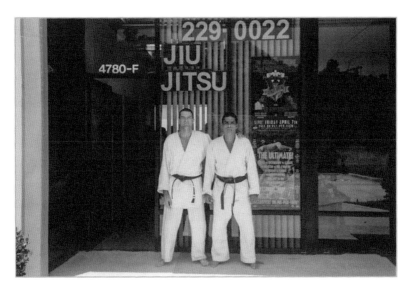

ALVARO ROMANO AND FABIO SANTOS IN SAN DIEGO, CA

CHAPTER 4

JIU-JITSU COMPETITIONS DURING THE 1970s and 1980s

The jiu-jitsu competitions were hotly disputed. Since only two representatives from each category represented the Gracie Gym, it was first necessary to complete an Eliminator Round with all students from the Gracie gyms that existed at the time.

These Eliminator Rounds took place at the Copacabana gym and the fighters alone already filled up the gym. They stood around the tatami mat and sat on the sides. There were dozens of people packed into a small space. Most of the time, Master Hélio Gracie and Master Carlos Gracie served as the judges and headed the fights.

During the 1970s, there were not many championships and once these competitions started to be organized, jiu-jitsu gained popularity. The creation of the Brazilian Confederation in Brazil and later the International Federation by Master Carlos Gracie Júnior was fundamental, since the organization of the Pan-American and global championships prompted the development of the sport. It became well known and the athletes earned visibility. Another important factor was the 1993 creation of the Ultimate Fighting Championship (UFC) by Master Rorion Gracie. I was at the first edition of this event in

Denver, when the world could witness the efficiency of jiu-jitsu with the fights by Royce Gracie. Rorion was responsible for enhancing the sport's popularity in the United States, with an entrepreneurial vision that helped create opportunities for the Brazilians to work with jiu-jitsu in the United States and worldwide.

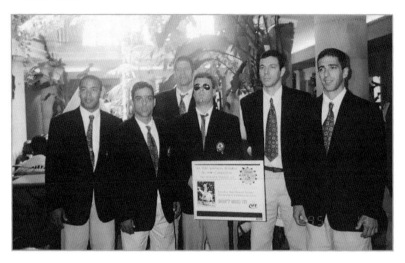

1995 FIRST JIU JITSU PAN AMERICAN BRAZILIAN DELEGATION. Left to right, Jose Alfredo (Doctor), Alvaro Romano (Physical Conditioner), Marcio Stambowsky and Rodrigo Miranda (Technical Coaches), Carlos Gracie Junior (President), Jose Henrique Teixeira (Vice President)

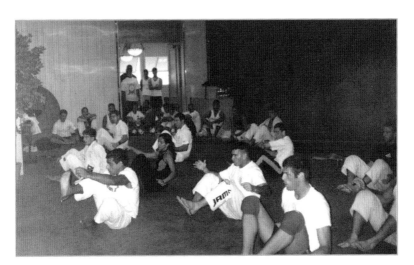

PROFESSOR ALVARO ROMANO TEACHING GINASTICA NATURAL CLASS TO BRAZILIAN TEAM

CHAPTER 5

HATHA YOGA AND THE BENEFITS FOR ATHLETES AND PRACTITIONERS

My first contact with Hatha Yoga was through the book by a Brazilian Master named Jose Hermógenes. This book sparked my interest in studying more about these Eastern techniques since I could understand the benefits, and primarily the spiritual part the author so heavily emphasized.

There were not many yoga styles in the 1980s. Hatha Yoga was the most popular, and in 1982, after the death of Rolls Gracie, I began to practice it at the gym of Professor Orlando Cani, in Rio de Janeiro. I recall that during this period, most students were older and had a different vision, since many people sought out yoga due to health issues and this proved the benefits of these techniques. I was the only jiu-jitsu fighter during the classes and as a Physical Education professional, it was not hard for me to understand the physiological effects of the breathing techniques and exercises that improved my flexibility, concentration and physical recovery. These included the stretches that already existed in the series I practice, created many, many years ago and which would later serve as an influence or were adapted from the different methods that would emerge.

In 1983, the first triathlon race including swimming, cycling and running was coming to Brazil and I thought it would be an important experience to participate in a long duration endurance race with characteristics that differed from the sports I practiced. I wanted to research the benefits of Hatha Yoga, how I could use breathing techniques and stretching to increase my endurance against fatigue from the training and improve my recovery.

For a race with a 1,500-meter (1-mile) swimming course, 60 kilometers (37 miles) of cycling and 14 kilometers (8.7 miles) of running, different training was required. I needed to practice these three types of sports, one after the other, just like it would be on race day. The training had to be as specific as possible, and this was a bit complicated due to the classes I had to give throughout the entire day. I had approximately 25 training days and because I didn't have the right bicycle for this type of competition, I tried to adapt my own training. I went to cycling classes and I tried to complete certain training sessions before the Hatha Yoga classes, since these helped me recover physically with breathing and stretching techniques, which I also used on the day of the event.

At the start of the swimming race with 400 competitors, I lost my goggles in all the commotion. It took me a great deal of effort to get away from the crowd and this tired me out. When I got out of the water at the end, I felt like I might faint. I was dizzy and seeing double. I was able to run slowly to the bicycle and when I started pedaling, I applied a breathing technique that helped me reduce the fatigue, leveling out my breaths and then using other techniques. However, I had only practiced before in a seated and motionless position, since I learned it during the series of classes. While on the bicycle, I continued to use different types of breathing, varying based on the difficulties I ran into. There were many other uphill parts and it was really hot. I started to recover and passed other competitors and ended up placing well. From the time I left the water until the finish line, I passed many people. I recovered during the race. This was an important experience for me to understand how these techniques really *can* make a difference and the importance of applying them when it comes to health and performance.

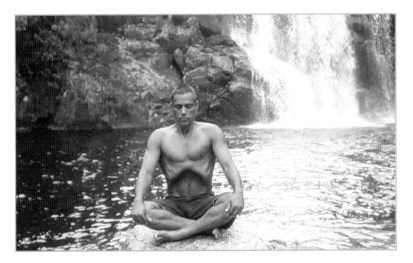

BREATHING TECHNIQUES

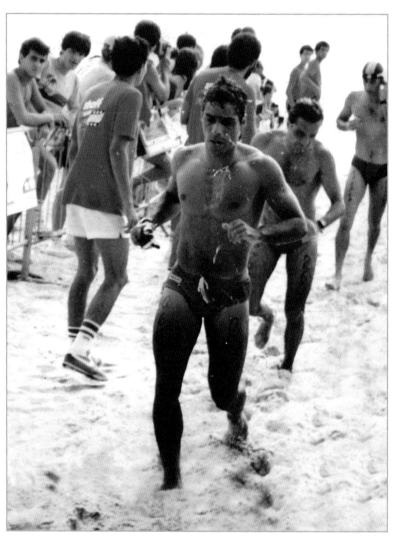

*1983, RIO DE JANEIRO, ALVARO ROMANO COMPETING IN
TRIATHLON*

CHAPTER 6

AN APPROACH TO THE IMPORTANCE OF SPECIFIC TRAINING

All types of training are important for physical preparation, but specific training has always been the priority in the work I undertook with athletes. There are sports like MMA, for which the athletes train in many different categories. And similarly to surfing, there is a lot of travel involved, plenty of injuries, a commitment to sponsors and many other factors that are a reality of these sports. Even though they get closer to professionalization each year, they are still determining the best way to organize and improve training.

As part of the specific training, athletes develop and improve the technique by practicing the sport, and that is when they obtain a more customized physical fitness.

Injuries and over-training have been known to weaken performance and many athletes' ability to consistently participate in competitions. This further leads to negative outcomes in their life, both in sports as well as financially.

Physical fitness should give athletes the conditions they need to develop their capacities to a maximum, and one detail that has always been very important is recovering from the physical and emotional toll of the training and competitions.

Since 1991, I have been part of a team with several fighters working as a physical trainer. We saw some very significant progress when the athletes, team and sponsors all perceived the importance of full-time training within a specified period of time for the competition we call CAMP. During CAMP, athletes can dedicate themselves the entire time solely and exclusively to their preparation for the event.

Scheduling the training involves factors such as the available time that the physical trainer has to work and the physical recovery from the training, which is a priority for me. An athlete who has recovered finishes the training always with the desire to train, and this is important in many aspects.

Often times, we think about what would be better: intensifying the preparation or emphasizing the recovery? These are questions that need to be analyzed, since there are several situations that need to be explored. This proved to be an interesting experience in my professional life, and in 1984, I began to observe these things when I went to work in the Physical Fitness area at Flamengo Yacht Club, home to one of Brazil's main soccer teams.

During my observation of the training agenda, I observed that we hardly had any days set aside for physical preparation. To better clarify, the following is a description of what the training was like:

Sunday:	Game
Monday:	Rest
Tuesday:	Sometimes there was physical training, which would be either a normal run or a circuit
Wednesday:	Technical training because the athletes could not train hard, since they had a game the next day
Thursday:	Game
Friday:	Rest
Saturday:	Light technical training because they had a game the next day

With little time to develop the physical aspect, the athletes built their endurance during the game itself. The training evolved and was modified increasingly more to add importance to the training known as regenerative or recovery training. Besides massages and sauna sessions, which were formally the basis of such work, the recovery training in the water, stretching exercises and several other techniques were implemented to help the athletes recover.

There are sports like MMA for which athletes train in several different sports types and have many different trainers. The physical trainer needs to be attentive during these training sessions, since many tend to use highly intense warm-ups during all sessions of the day, which really tires the athletes out. The ideal solution is for the physical trainer to be the one who is always responsible for the warm-ups, since it is he or she who prepares the athlete to start the session for any type of sport type that is trained, leading the coach directly to the specific training. If each trainer from a sport type makes the athlete do intense warm-ups, then this athlete will not have his or her ideal performance. This is a common issue in MMA.

To better understand the importance of the recovery training, here is an example of a weekly training schedule for MMA athletes:

Sunday:	Rest
Monday:	Morning – boxing; Afternoon – jiu-jitsu
Tuesday:	Morning– muay thai; Afternoon – specific jiu-jitsu training; positions and drops
Wednesday:	Morning – resting or light recovery and/or mobility training; Afternoon – sparring
Thursday:	Morning – wrestling; Afternoon – specific training of positions and techniques to be used, depending on the adversary's characteristics
Friday:	Morning – jiu-jitsu; Afternoon – boxing
Saturday:	Sparring

Observations: The training is varied similarly to boxing. One day, there is combat school, while on another, gauntlet training, just like jiu-jitsu training sessions.

It is important to observe the athlete's physical wear and the importance of recovery training. Many times, this training is done during the warm-up before the training session using breathing techniques and joint mobility exercises.

The physical trainer needs to have the knowledge to demonstrate the recovery training at all training sites, since we need to optimize the time as much as possible due to the need for rest between morning and afternoon training sessions.

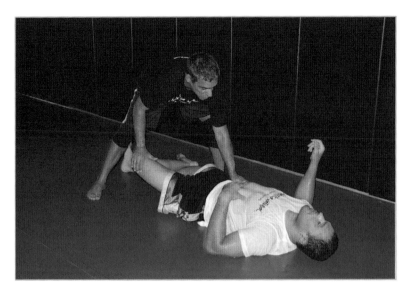

PROFESSOR ALVARO ROMANO TEACHING RECOVERY TRAINING WITH BREATHING TECHNIQUES AND STRETCHING TO FIGHTER RODRIGO "MINOTAURO" NOGUEIRA

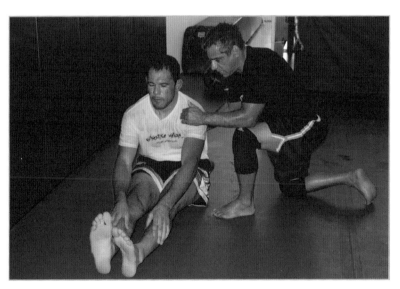

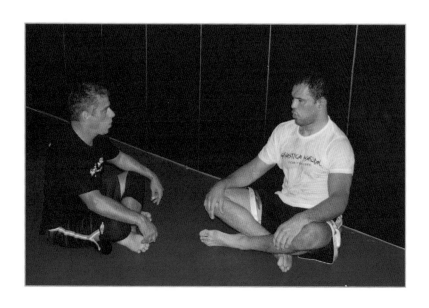

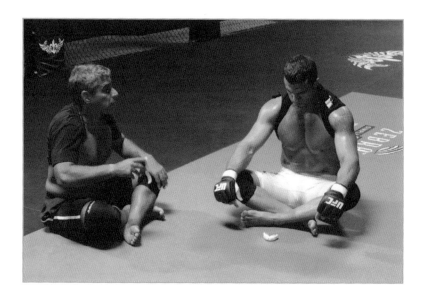

PROFESSOR ALVARO ROMANO TEACHING THE FIGHTER VITOR BELFORT FOR UFC IN LAS VEGAS

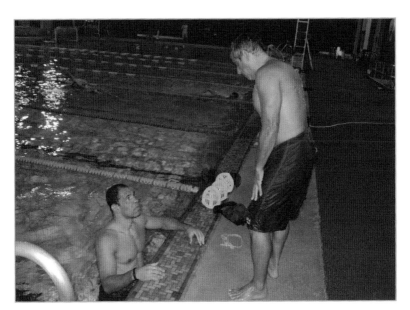

PROFESSOR ALVARO ROMANO AND ROGERIO "MINOTOURO" NOGUEIRA RECOVERY TRAINING IN THE POOL, SAN DIEGO, CA

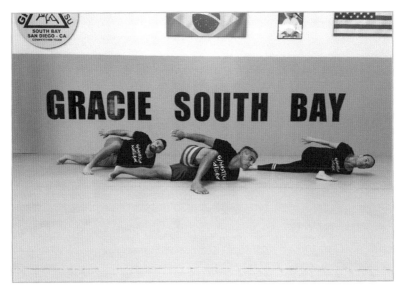

PROFESSOR ALVARO ROMANO TEACHING THE FIGHTERS FABRÍCIO CAMÕES AND LETICIA RIBEIRO

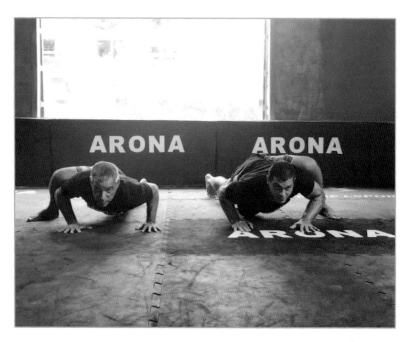

GINASTICA NATURAL TRAINING SESSION WITH THE FIGHTER RICARDO ARONA

SURFING

For surfing, the circuit is tiring, since there is lots of travel and the athlete generally goes alone. That is why an evaluation and adequate training before starting the circuit can prevent injuries. Furthermore, during the circuit it is ideal to include maintenance and recovery training, since the priority for developing performance and improving technique will always be to practice the sport itself in the different conditions that will be found at the competition sites.

For any sport, it is ideal to work with a multidisciplinary team, including a physical trainer, physician, psychologist, nutritionist and physical therapist.

At the end of the competitions, certain factors are important. These include:

1) Physical and psychological evaluation of the athlete, with meetings to evaluate what was done in the past and what can be improved;

2) Consultations with physicians, physical therapists and nutritionists so that they can all complete an evaluation based on their respective specialty and listen to the athlete's feedback, since this is something very important we need always to move forward;

3) Evaluate whether the athlete needs to continue with the physical therapy and balance this work with the weightlifting, cardio and preparation training so the body can withstand the harder workouts during the specific training period;

4) It is important to add that this training is not very intense, but rather more of a maintenance training that may become more intense since there is always a possibility that another event may be scheduled;

5) During this period, leisure and rest are important. However, the athlete needs to have an "athlete's holiday" and a good strategy. What many choose are activities or sports that do not cause injuries and are done in a recreational way, like swimming, surfing, hiking – something outdoors and pleasurable;

6) Depending on the sport type chosen during this phase, it is important to suggest activities that extend beyond the normal work environments. One example is the MMA athletes, who spend most or nearly all of their time inside closed environments. In their case, outdoor activities are a good option.

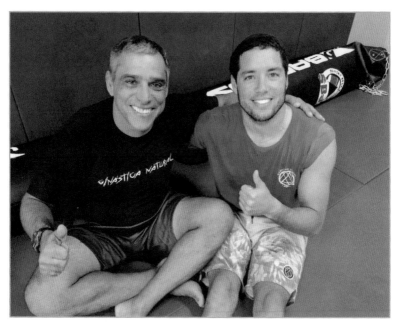

AFTER TRAINING SECTION IN HAWAII WITH WORLD CHAMPION ADRIANO "MINEIRINHO" SOUZA

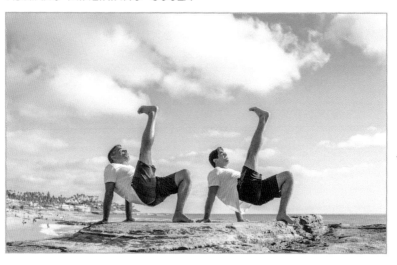

GINASTICA NATURAL EXERCISE FOR SURFING

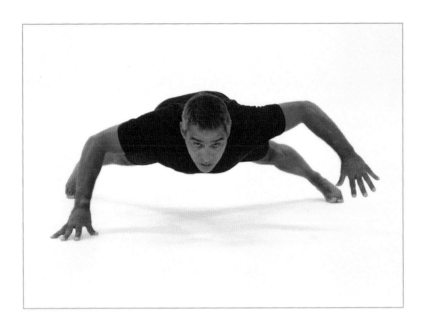

GINASTICA NATURAL ADVANCED EXERCISE 1

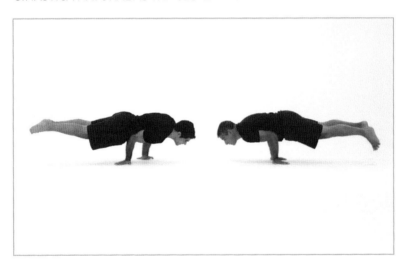

2

CHAPTER 7

SOME IMPORTANT ASPECTS DURING THE PHASES OF PHYSICAL AND PSYCHOLOGICAL PREPARATION

Psychological preparation is a decisive factor and the most important of all, observing details that often go unnoticed and which are many times decisive. Some believe the gain is small. However, for a high-performance sport, even the smallest gain can be decisive. It can be the one to make the difference, since the level goes up each day. Everyone completes the training, studies their adversaries and learns about techniques that are often the specialty of just a few. Certain precautions can help, such as:

1) DURING THE TRAINING

During the training phase, it is important to observe the learning factor, the new techniques being taught or what can be done to improve. Accordingly, the trainer-athlete and athlete-athlete relationship is quite important. The MMA training in general involves the participation of several athletes from different categories who are invited to assist with these training sessions. Some are still unknown and it is necessary to make them understand that they are there to assist and may even discover an opportunity in the future. However, to make this happen, they need to follow the trainers' recommendations, have a good attitude with the athlete they will fight and work to ensure that they make the most of their performance, but with peace of mind and not getting involved in a personal competition.

There have been situations in which the invited athlete unintentionally injures the main athlete simply because he or she gets carried away. This is something very important to be observed by the trainers so they can correct the athlete at the right time.

2) DURING TRAINING PERIODS

Evaluate the conditions to always achieve top performance and improve the technical, physical, psychological and social aspects.

The site where the training will take place and the conditions of this training are crucial. There needs to be an appropriate place to train each category, without the risk for accidents. These are all important details. There have been situations in which an athlete with a scheduled fight gets cut on a piece of glass from a window located near the training site and then the fight has to be cancelled. Therefore, it is essential that the sites have infrastructure that is completely safe, and if possible, a site for physical therapy and recovery training.

A training site that is located near the site where the athletes are staying is important so they can avoid long travels and be able to rest and recover. Meals should be planned so that the athletes does not have to go long periods without eating after training and the entire team should be able to get to the training sites without too much inconvenience for the athlete due to long wait times or delays.

3) TRANSPORTATION

The goal is to establish measures that can prevent a less-than-optimal performance. The trips are tiring, the time zone is often different and affects the athlete's performance, and this needs to be controlled. The scheduling of the trip should be well planned, as well as the arrival of the athlete and the specific training used to help them recover from the trip and time zone difference. This planning should extend to the trip for the whole team.

4) DURING THE COMPETITIONS

This is the most important day, so it is necessary to prevent and control all factors that can reduce or negatively affect the athlete's ability to achieve their best result. These include preventing too many people who are not part of the training team from coming into contact with the athlete, especially if they can get them overly excited or wear them out. The ideal solution is to have the person responsible control the number of people in contact with the athlete. People who are not part of the team and who may negatively affect the athlete's concentration should be totally blocked. From the moment the athlete wakes up to the time of their fight, they should be in a peaceful place they can trust.

Having participated as a physical trainer during important events around the world, I can confirm that the psychological aspect on the days preceding the competition and during the final moments is what may determine the success of the effort made.

There are athletes who are not very well prepared, and on the day of the competition, they do not perform as expected and they have the sensation that they did not do their best. There are also others who do not train as much or those who end up replacing someone who is hurt at the last minute and actually perform very well.

The psychological factor has a major influence during preparation and certain techniques and observations can help athletes achieve better results, such as evaluating anxious behaviors, pre-competition stress and factors that may influence the results. This can vary from one athlete to the next. An extroverted athlete, for example, is different than an introverted one. One may have a harder time concentrating than another, and this is why we need to study this behavior during the training period so that on the days leading up to the competition, we will know exactly which techniques to use.

Since 1991, when they restarted the free-for-all events in Brazil, I began using these techniques to control anxiety and stress. They are breathing techniques that promote physical and mental relaxation. Controlled breathing directly improves one's ability to concentrate.

These techniques need to be well applied, since specific breathing needs to be used at different times, paired with relaxation techniques that many mistakenly use before the competition starts, negatively affecting their performance.

A technique that should be used during the week preceding the competition and which may help control anxious behavior is mental training, which involves motivation, reinforcement of self-confidence, emotional control, concentration and several other factors. The pressure that many athletes feel during the competitions may elevate the stress level and this varies for each athlete. We can apply a simulation technique and mentally reproduce the elements and behaviors present during the competition that can weaken the athlete's ideal performance. This exercise can be applied at the end of each training session one week before the competition, and consists of reproducing all situations that normally occur on the day of the fight.

This technique can be applied with the athlete lying down in a comfortable position and focusing on abdominal breathing – inhaling slowly to dilate the abdomen exhaling to slowly contract the abdomen.

After about five minutes, the trainer, using a calm voice, begins to verbally reproduce the situations from the day of the fight for the athlete to visualize. These include the time the athlete wakes up, getting the material ready to go to the fight, leaving the hotel, the trip and arrival to the site of the event, heading to the locker room, warming up, entering the competition site and all phases until visualizing the fight and victory.

This visualization may be repeated several times and it's interesting to observe that based on how you talk, depending on the situation, the athlete's heart rate may either increase or decrease. For example, this may happen when the athlete visualizes his or her entry into the stadium.

I developed this technique with several athletes during many competitions, but a specific situation of when it truly made a difference was for the fight of athlete Rodrigo Minotaur against Randy Couture during UFC 102 in Portland, Oregon.

We completed the training in San Diego, California, and during a conversation with some people, I found out that the local fans were mostly all rooting for the adversary. During the mental training completed weeks before the fight, I always addressed this detail. When visualizing his entrance into the gymnasium, I always asked the athlete to imagine the adversary's fans, to imagine them booing, and I noticed that during the first days when I mentioned this situation, the athlete's heart rate changed a little and over time slowed down. On the day of the fight, the athlete did exactly what we had trained. After the fight, I was close by when a reporter from a Brazilian show asked him if he was feeling pressure during that situation and he responded that it was easy, that he had trained the same situation over and over and that when it actually occurred, he was able to reduce the pressure.

CHAPTER 8

PARTS OF A TRAINING SESSION

A training session consists of the following:
Preparatory Part - Main Part - Final Part

Preparatory Part:

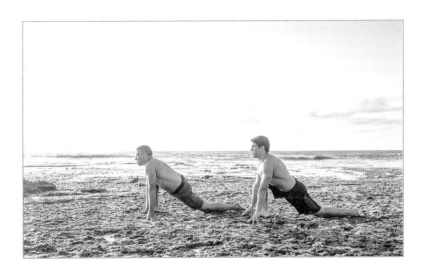

Designed to explain what will be done during the training session, what the training will be like, and at the same time, motivate the athlete for the tasks that will be completed following the warm-up, which is a very important phase.

Besides its purpose of shifting the athlete's body from a resting state to an active one, we can also use it to prevent injuries and offer the athlete perfect conditions to complete the tasks. We need approximately 3-5 minutes after starting the work for the body to shift from the resting state to the proper state for mobilization and coordination. This is because the human system does not function immediately as the level of the activity grows.

There are many cases of athletes who, without a proper warm-up, can reach the end of the competition without being able to perform to their full potential.

The warm-up for training may last approximately 20-40 minutes, and during the competition, the warm-up can start up to 1:30 hours ahead of time. In both cases, the athlete should use mobility exercises, movements that simulate those of the competition and stimuli for psychological preparation. The trainer should be attentive to always keep the athlete motivated and vary the warm-up routine. Shorter and faster movements should be used to stimulate the reaction time, but only approaching maximum effort, combined with active rest and breathing techniques.

GINASTICA NATURAL EXERCISES FOR WARM UP

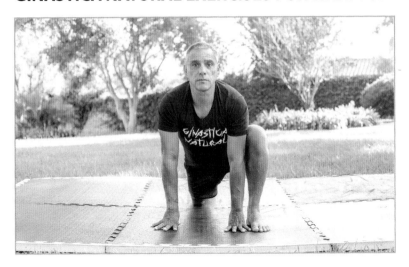

QUADRICEPS STRETCHING

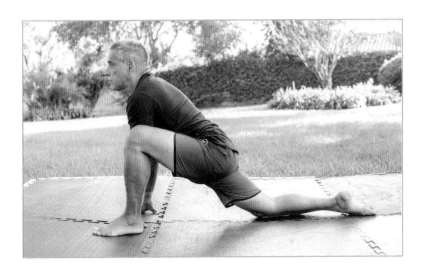

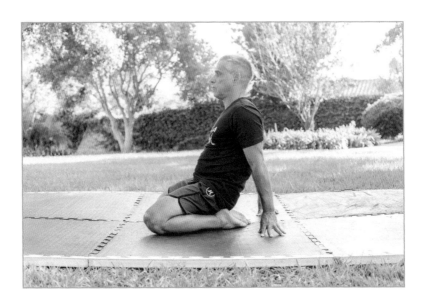

HANDS BACK HIPS UP 1

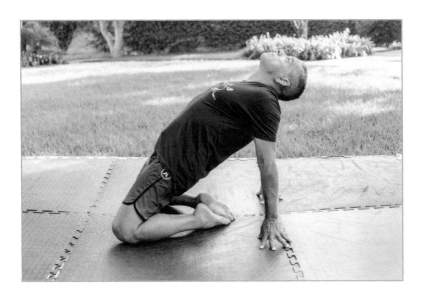

HANDS BACK HIPS UP 2

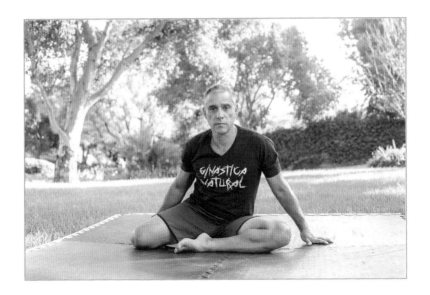

GINASTICA NATURAL HIPS SCAPE 1

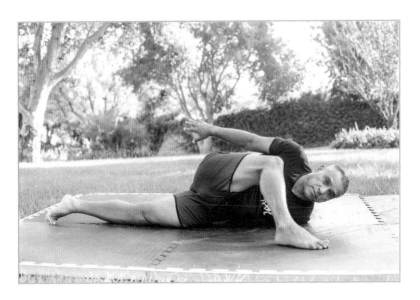

2

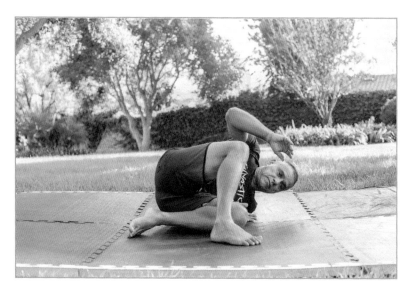

3

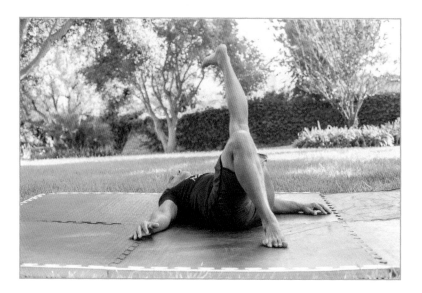

4

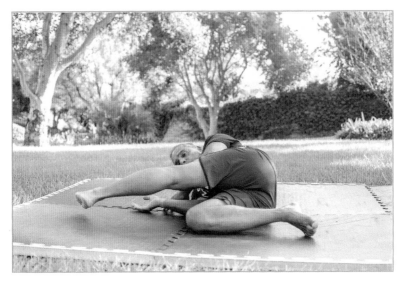

5

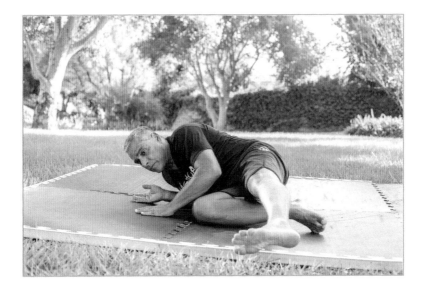

6

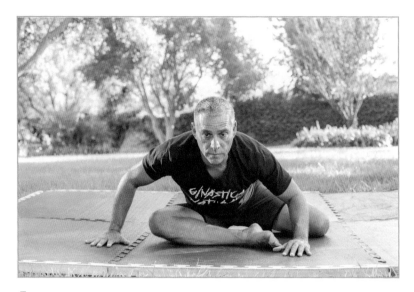

7

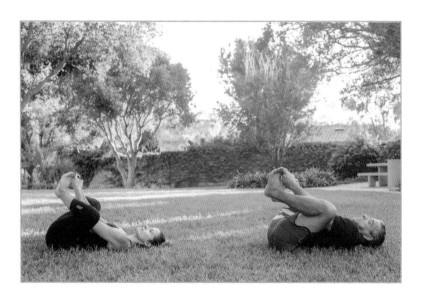

MONKEY STRETCH 1

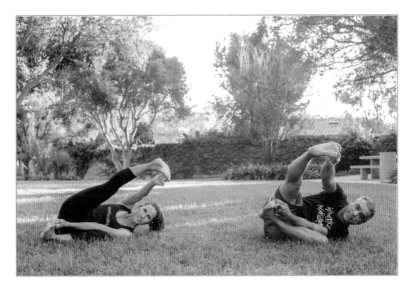

2

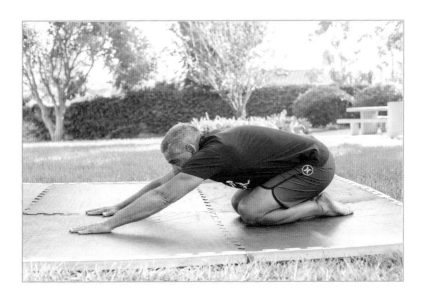

DIVING MOVEMENT 1

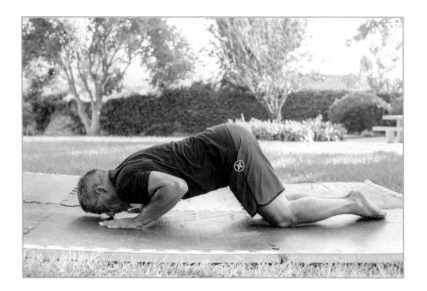

2

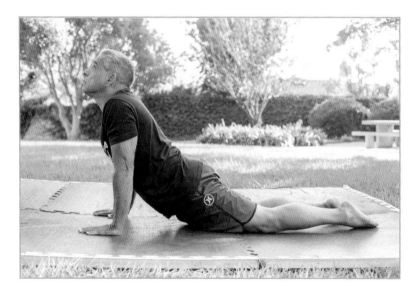

3

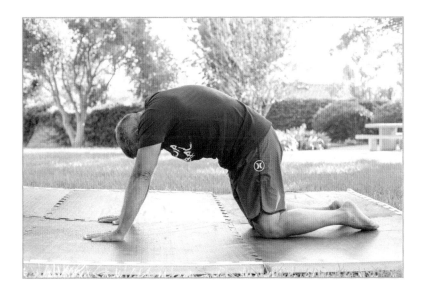

4

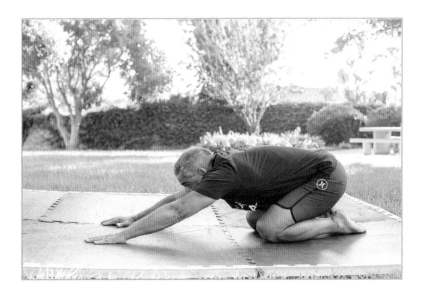

5

Main part:

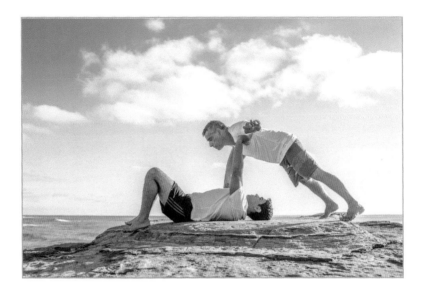

This would be the technical and specific training to reproduce all situations typically found in the competition.

Observation: For surfing, which depends on the conditions of the ocean, specific training can be used on calm days or in the pool, which can be used to reproduce the situations found when practicing the sport.

The functional training is important and is being used by several trainers. However, it is worth noting that this training aims to reproduce the movements of the sport practiced. The thing is, when the athletes practice the sport, they already overwork certain joints, such as during surfing with their increasingly radical moves that have a major impact and involve lots of twists. It is interesting to observe that many athletes do not have satisfactory muscle balance due precisely to these moves, since they are surfing with an even greater strain on one of the legs and trying to reproduce these moves with the same exercises like jumps or high-impact workouts during this functional training without first working on this muscle balance with specific exercises. This lack of balance may have a negative effect on the athlete, making him or her more predisposed to injuries.

GINASTICA NATURAL EXERCISES
UPPER BODY/LEGS

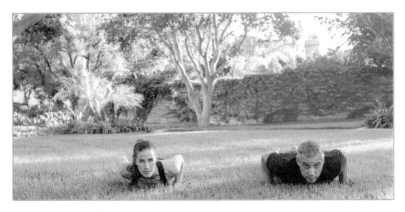

CROSS PUSH UP 1

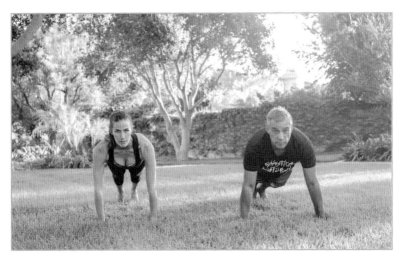

2

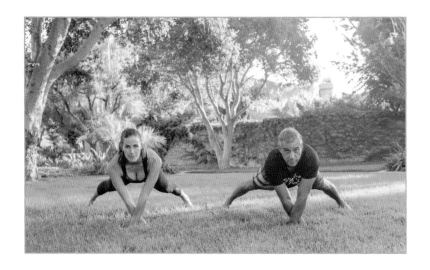

3

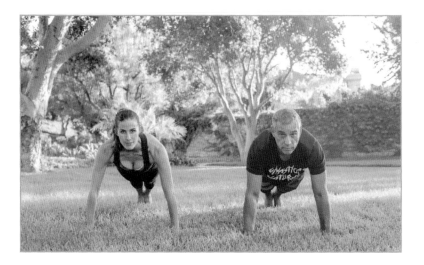

4

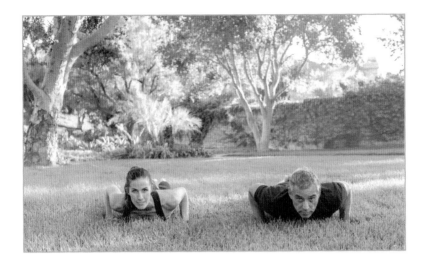

5

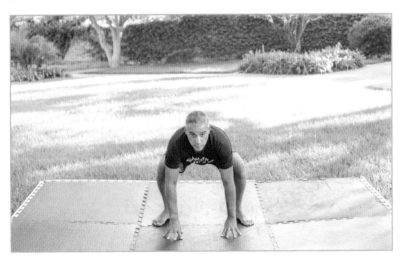

FRONT KICK 1

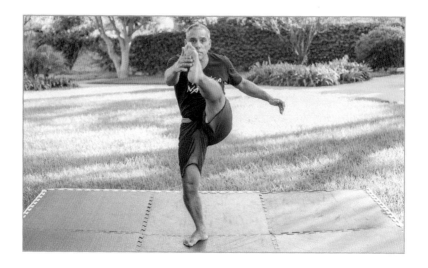

2

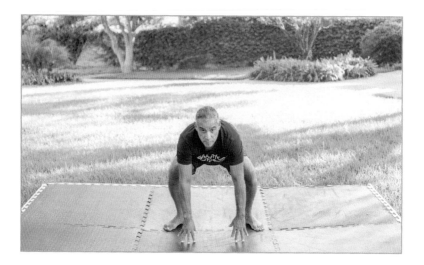

3

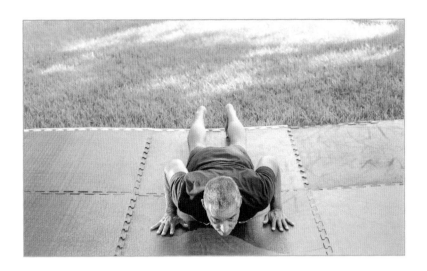

ADVANCED PUSH UP 1

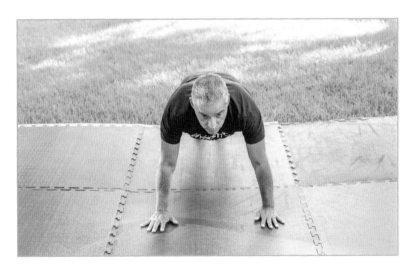

2

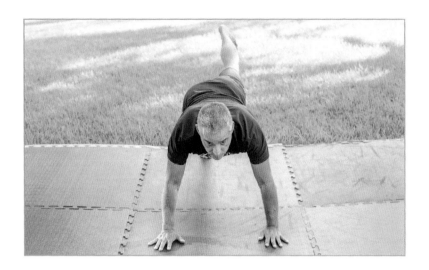

3

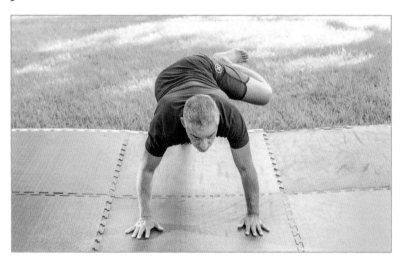

4

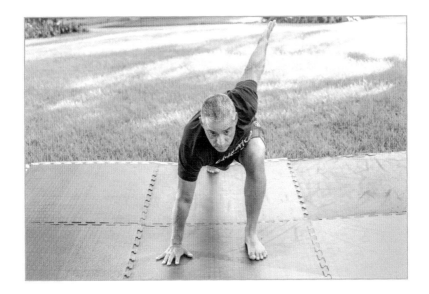

5

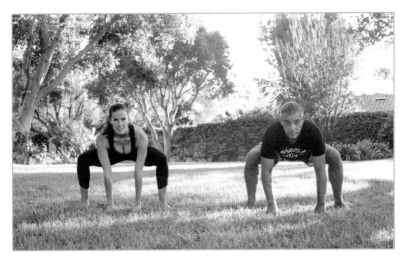

LATERAL MONKEY 1

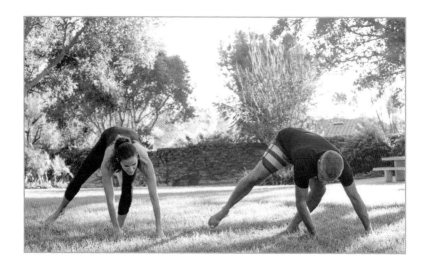

2

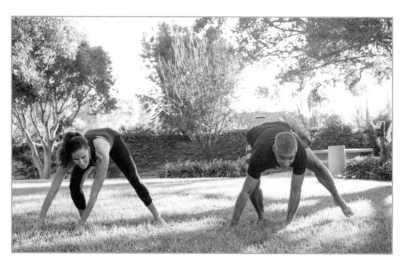

3

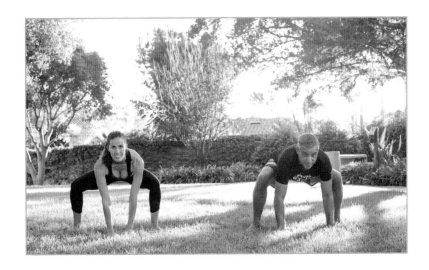

4

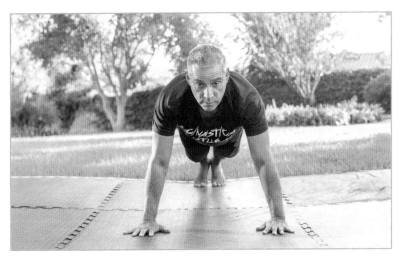

SPIDER PUSH UP 1

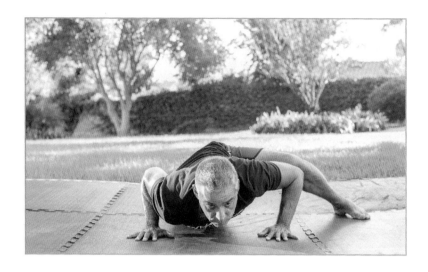

2

GINASTICA NATURAL ABS EXERCISE:

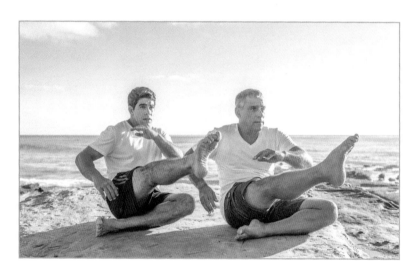

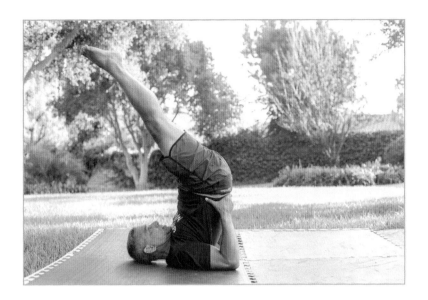

GINASTICA NATURAL CANDLE ABS 1

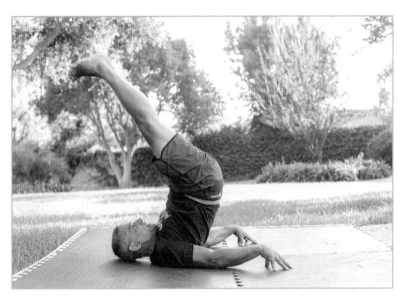

2

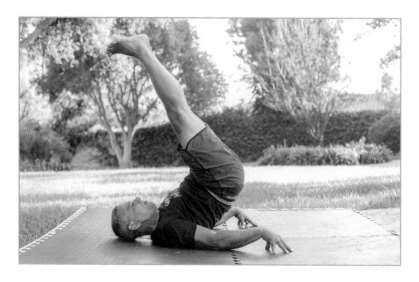

3

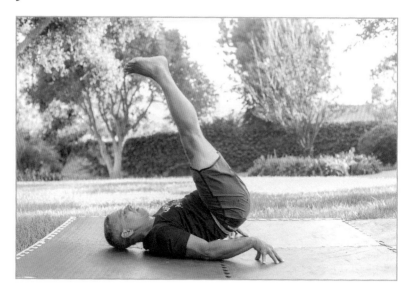

4

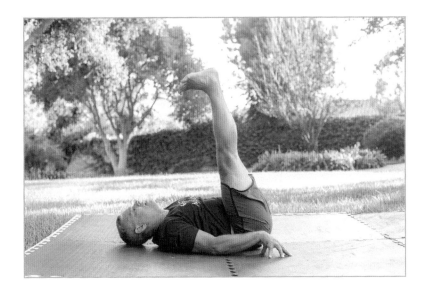

5

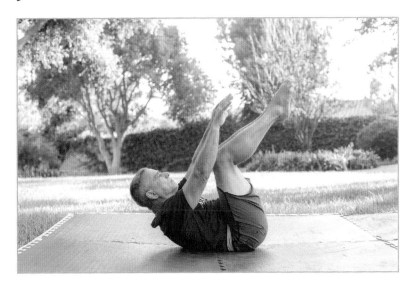

6

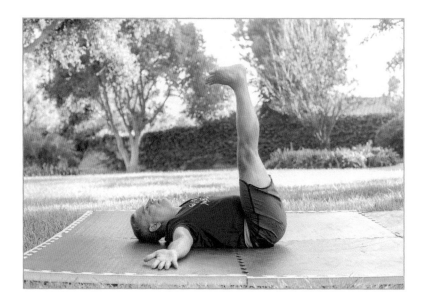

7

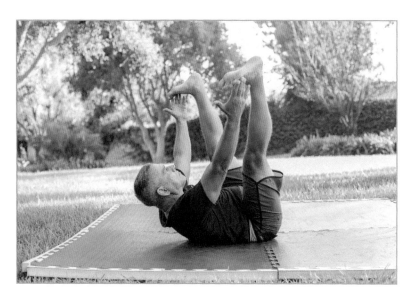

8

Final part:

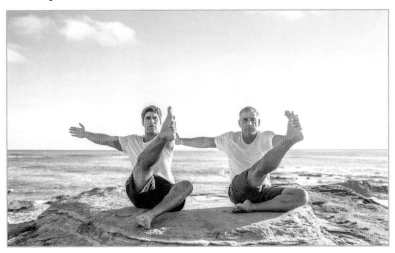

A very important phase that heavily influences performance. The ideal solution is for an athlete to finish the training always with the desire to continue so that on the next day, he or she can have a good performance. That is why we need to help the athlete recover from all of the effort made while training during the main phase, since this is generally associated with a high level of physical and emotional stress. To begin the recovery phase, try to work with joint mobility exercises at a calm and moderate pace for between 10 and 15 minutes and then do some breathing and relaxation techniques. These will help more quickly eliminate lactic acid, consequently helping the athlete recover.

GINASTICA NATURAL EXERCISE FOR RECOVERY

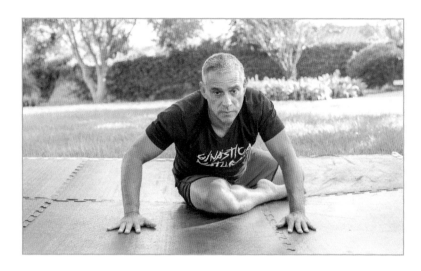

BASIC ROLL 1

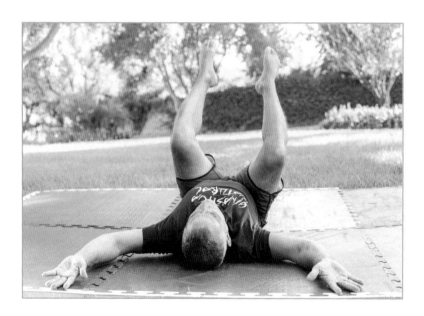

2

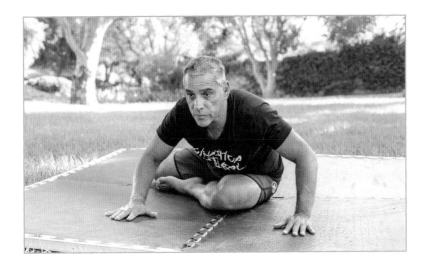

3

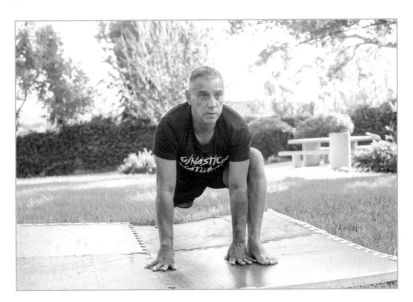

ADVANCED ROLL 1

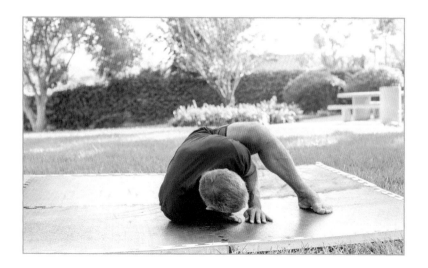

2

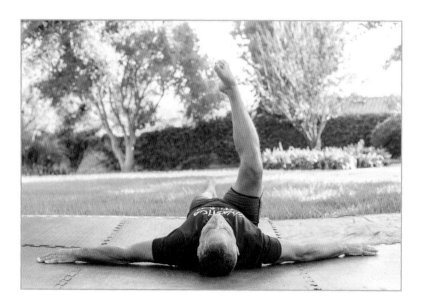

3

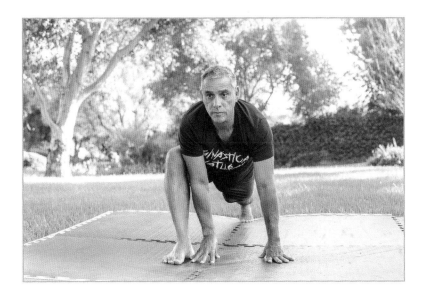

4

CHAPTER 9

BREATHING TECHNIQUES

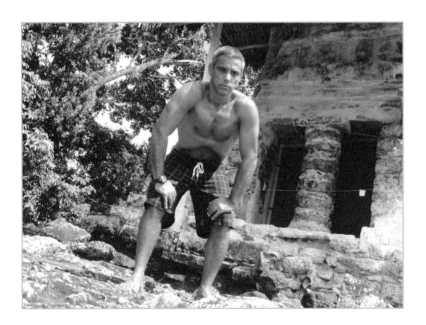

These techniques have been developed for thousands of years. Understanding and knowing how to breathe can transform our life in many aspects. Breathing is the only physiological process that is both voluntary and involuntary. If we want, we can control our breathing: speed it up, slow it down, stop it, restart it. There are several techniques for controlling and being aware of our breathing, such as slowly and controlled or more vigorously. These techniques strengthen the diaphragm, the deep musculature that is important for stabilizing our body, promoting well-being, health and quality of life, so much so that they are considered by yoga masters and gurus to be purification techniques due to the physiological benefits they offer.

The vital capacity is a person's overall capacity to inhale and exhale and is evaluated based on the power of the respiratory muscles and elastic resistance of the chest wall and lungs for expansion and contraction. We generally find it easier to test the power of our breathing by blowing air out vigorously. However, another good exercise is to breathe slowly, inhaling gradually and using the entire range of the breathing movement, beginning with the diaphragm, back area and then sub-clavicle area, to then exhale slowly trying to prolong this process to the maximum. If we try to reverse it – begin with the chest, then ribs and finally, the abdomen – it is normal to find this more difficult, since we generally breathe only in the chest part, which leads to short, fast breathing.

By practicing breathing techniques, we can expand breathing movements, and consequently, our vital capacity, since the abdominal muscles will move the diaphragm, intensifying its activity in both directions and at the maximum extension levels, widely expanding the capacity of the thorax.

Correct breathing is very important for our health, and for athletes, it heavily influences performance. By applying these techniques for over 30 years with athletes from different types of sports, we have seen some excellent results when applying it before, during and after training. Correct breathing during training increases endurance against fatigue and several different studies prove its effectiveness in terms of emotional control, the faster processing of information, improved concentration and control of anxiety and stress.

ABDOMINAL OR DIAPHRAGM BREATHING

In 1982, I began to practice breathing techniques and better understand their physiological effects on the organism and importance for everyone seeking a healthy lifestyle. In the beginning, it is normal to experience difficulty. However, everyone can do it progressively, starting with slow, deep abdominal breathing.

We use abdominal breathing when we sleep, which is a time of deep relaxation, although involuntary. It is ideal that we practice this technique consciously during other hours of our day as well.

Follow these steps to practice abdominal breathing:

Seated and with your legs crossed – or if you have a hard time sitting in this position, you can lean up against a wall – lie down with your legs bent and gently place your hands over your abdomen.

With your eyes closed, try to inhale by slowing dilating the abdomen and when you exhale, gently contract it. Work to gradually increase the breathing in and out, always slow and smooth.

Practice this technique for about 20 minutes twice a day to later try out more advanced techniques. At the end of each session, you will experience a sensation of calm and relaxation. In the beginning, you may have some difficulty breathing 100% abdominally, but you will find that you achieve this control little by little. Some people have a hard time concentrating. They start thinking about other things. If this happens, simply re-focus on the breathing itself. Even if you find this happening several times, continue because with training, you will increasingly be able to keep your focus on the abdominal breathing.

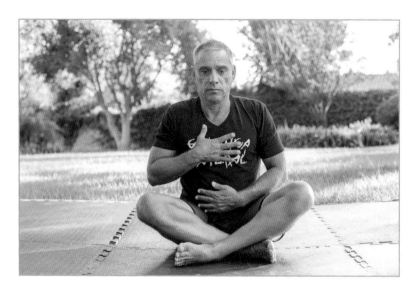

POSITION FOR DIAPHRAGM BREATHING

ILIOCOSTALIS (RIBS) BREATHING

There is a connection between abdominal and iliocostalis breathing. To practice this type of breathing, place the tip of the fingers on the sides of the ribs while breathing in slowly, expanding the movement of the ribs to the sides and increasing the breathing movement. Then, exhale while trying to inhale and exhale each time more and expand the movements to the sides, without breathing through the chest.

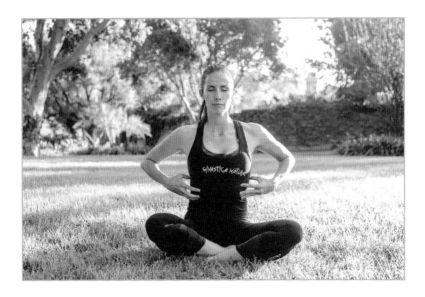

POSITION FOR ILIOCOSTALIS (RIBS) BREATHING

COMPLETE BREATHING

Complete breathing is when we join abdominal, iliocostalis and now sub-clavicular (chest) breathing.

For this technique, the best position is seated with your legs crossed. Close your eyes and try to inhale slowly and gently through your nose, beginning with abdominal breathing, then onto iliocostalis and finally sub-clavicular breathing. If you want, you may stop breathing for a few seconds and when you exhale, start the opposite way: inhale first through the chest, then iliocostalis and then finally abdominal. With this technique, you can exhale through the mouth as if blowing out a candle, exhaling out the air very slowly and making this process last as long as possible. Another option is to blow the air out through your nose during this same process, slowly and gently, remaining fully focused on the technique.

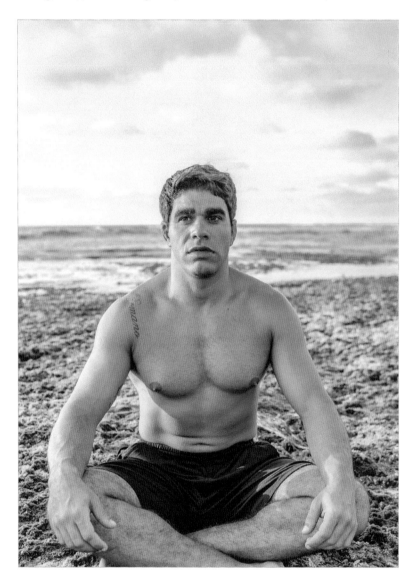

POSITION FOR COMPLETE BREATHIMG

ABDOMINAL SELF-MASSAGE

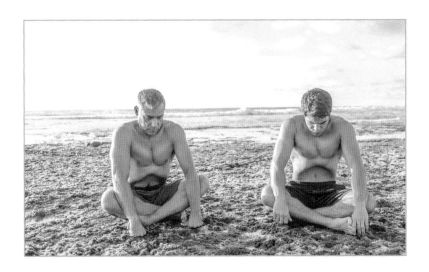

Because it is more advanced, this technique should be practiced by people who already have a basic understanding of breathing techniques. It offers several benefits and a sensation of well-being and calm. It is a technique that demands a high level of concentration and control. One of the benefits of this technique is its effectiveness combating back aches and discomfort in the lower back, since moving the diaphragm in different directions and its connection with the lower back vertebrae and deep musculature helps stretch the back and relaxes the lower back muscles. For this technique, sit with your legs crossed and hands resting in front. Begin with a few slow abdominal breaths and then exhale more rigorously by contracting the abdomen. Hold your breath and try to suck in your abdominal region for a few seconds and then inhale slowly. Repeat this several times or breathe a few more times between one massage and another, if you need to. The idea is to suck in the abdominal region more each time.

Try not to do this movement in an isolated fashion, but rather in alignment with the rest of the body, feeling your entire torso move.

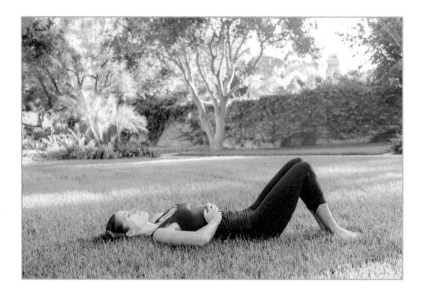

OPTIONAL POSITION FOR ABDOMINAL BREATHING AND RELAXATION

CHAPTER 10

TRAINING AND BREATHING

It is also very important to control breathing while exercising or in the event of some uncomfortable situation that emerges during training and competitions, since by being aware of our breathing at this moment, we will have improved endurance against fatigue.

Notice the trend of many athletes and others who practice physical activity to inhale whenever they make any movement, holding their breath and contracting several different parts of the body that are often not even being used. Controlling your breathing while in movement helps you achieve a unique level of relaxation, a very important physical quality that involves relaxing those muscles that are not being used during the completion of an exercise. One example would be to do an abdominal exercise and contract the muscles of the face. Breathing while in movement is presumably natural, but once we start to increase the intensity of the effort, we also increase the production of carbon gas, which is responsible for the sensation of fatigue. When we release the first carbon gas, we facilitate the entry of oxygen, which will improve our recovery. However, to achieve this we need to exhale and release the air, primarily if we are tired and out of breath.

Breathing is important even during a less intense activity, such as stretching and flexibility training. If when stretching out you work harmoniously, exhaling when you are curved and inhaling slowly when you are holding he stretch, you will feel more comfortable and relaxed and, accordingly, you will be able to go further.

CHAPTER 11

THE *GINASTICA NATURAL* METHOD

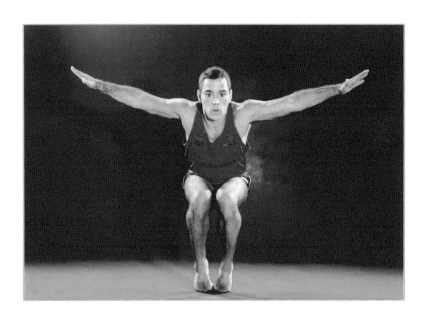

The History and Empirical Base of
Ginastica Natural

In order to develop any method, you must practice, study and apply it, and after many years of quantitative research, it is possible to plan and elaborate a methodology to be applied in different areas of human movement.

Technology has made it easier to transmit information, and each day, we see methods created from books, videos or the Internet that have not been practiced long enough to be developed safely by practitioners. *Ginastica Natural*, which began empirically, required many years to achieve its due recognition.

The video and photo archives and all the historical material showing the elaboration and evolution of the method have proven it was a slow, gradual process before reaching where we are today.

For the students completing courses around the world, I always try to clarify that success does not come only during normal practice. You must go the "extra mile," and this is only possible with hard work and dedication.

For the classes that I gave at the university, I debated with my students about the reason they all needed to learn the same content in the same way. When they started out professionally, some were successful and others gave up on their profession. I explained that this was due to the way that each one of them understands what was taught, how it will be applied, and primarily, the extra time that they will dedicate to testing it out, improving it and adapting it.

When developing something new, you cannot tread the known path by copying or doing something that has been done. People are unique, they have different characteristics, and it is important for us to listen to our intuition when it comes to our ideas. We need dedication and discipline for theoretical and practical studies.

We are always learning, and transformation is a characteristic of human beings. This is the only way we can develop methods and concepts. The main characteristic of science is constant progress.

My personal life has had a major influence in prompting me to develop *Ginastica Natural*. Outdoor exercises and those that use the weight of the body itself were part of my entire athletic development. Being born in a suburb of Rio de Janeiro, childhood games were part of this development: playing soccer on the streets, climbing trees, running, etc. When I moved to Ipanema, which is located near Arpoador Beach, a major surfing hub in Rio de Janeiro, I was already a teenager and began to surf, play beach soccer, capoeira, swim in the ocean and practice jiu-jitsu. The neuromuscular training was limited, since there were no workout stations on the beach like you see in gyms today. Our strength training was on the bars installed on the sands of the beach. When I joined the University in the area of Physical Education, it was pretty much focused on sports like volleyball, soccer and basketball, although with very high quality content in the area of motor skill learning, psychomotricity and performance training, and all of us professors had to be creative. Without modern equipment, the functional training and that using the weight of the body itself were applied in different areas of Physical Education. At the time, my thoughts as a professor were already on teaching my students these natural exercise concepts, activities in contact with nature and sports.

Training for approximately four hours a day, I tested out all the exercises first to only then teach them after. These represented important phases for developing the methodology that is constantly perfected, such as the following described below:

WITH RELATION TO THE PRACTITIONER AND METHOD

❶ Viewing / Questioning / Experimentation

When presenting something new, we will always have questions and doubts. Some students were hesitant about taking part in the classes due to the difficulty they had completing certain movements associated with body awareness that *Ginastica Natural* demands of its practitioners. Generally, when people have a hard time completing some technique, they do not train and seek to improve, but rather continue with those techniques they are able to do. Stretching and flexibility, which are the physical qualities developed in *Ginastica Natural*, have always been cited by many as a reason for not participating in classes. However, the opposite is ideal, since we need to work precisely those areas we need to improve, and trying out a class is the best way to understand what *Ginastica Natural* is all about.

❷ The practice itself / experience of the body movements / memorization of the movements / learning

Practice all the movements, experience them, learn and evaluate. This was necessary for improving and researching a way to teach these movements with a methodology that could facilitate the students' learning and ensure they did the exercises effectively.

❸ Experimentation with control / evaluation of the context and development of motor patterns / application of new stimuli

Starting from the time that the exercises were developed, they were applied in a group setting for experimentation and evaluation. These groups included mostly martial arts and surfer athletes, which allowed us to work safely, since they had the physical conditions to try out the exercises and offer us important feedback to make the necessary adaptations for beginner students. The outdoor classes at beaches and parks in Rio de Janeiro attracted lots of practitioners, who disseminated what they learned and helped motivate people who were seeking a unique and innovative training type. At the gym, we also used music during the classes.

❹ The *Ginastica Natural* method / systemization of knowledge / conceptualization and systematization of new knowledge

Besides the systemization of the exercises developed during the training and methodology of the classes, the joint work with professionals from the physical therapy area has helped increase knowledge and understanding of *Ginastica Natural*, which besides serving as a method for physical training, quality of life, health and wellness, can also prevent injuries and help with rehabilitation.

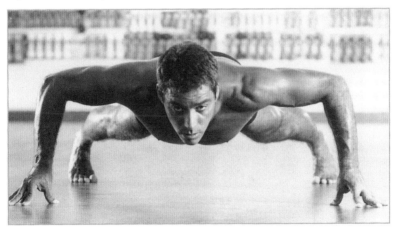

PROFESSOR ALVARO ROMANO IN 1991 PRACTICING GINASTICA SPIDER PUSH UP

CHAPTER 12

PHYSICAL EDUCATION AND ITS POSSIBILITIES

Physical Education offers us a range of possibilities to work with. For a professional to develop something new and be able to effectively implement his or her ideas, it is important to study and work in the different areas of the profession. In my case, working with children was important and a major source of learning. It was my first job as a Physical Education professor at a holiday camp for kids, held in 1977 with Jose Henrique Leão, a friend and fellow professor. This project was different than the others at the time. We took the kids to a ranch in a small town located in the mountains of Rio de Janeiro to spend a weekend or the entire week. During this time, we focused on an introduction to sports, together with work that could offer everyone the opportunity to practice physical activity and motivate them, and for those who expressed interest, recommend a specific activity for more advanced training.

In 1978, I began a project to offer classes on the beaches of Rio de Janeiro, where we trained using the weight of the body itself and materials like rope and cones, together with a circuit course. This is known today as functional training.

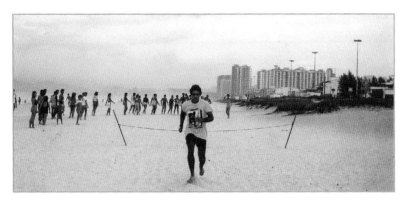

BEACH TRAINING IN RIO DE JANEIRO, 1982

In 1984, I organized the first surfing course in Rio de Janeiro for children and adolescents, including the basics on the physical preparation for the sport.

The name *"Ginastica Natural"* emerged sometime after I had started using this class model. In the beginning, when I began giving the classes at Latin America's largest chain of gyms in Rio de Janeiro, these classes were known as "Body Movement."

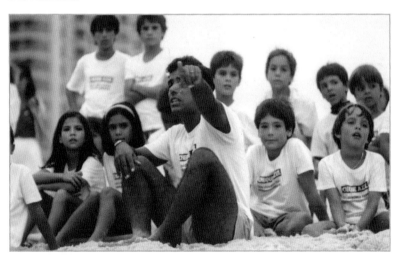

SURFING COURSE IN RIO DE JANEIRO, 1984

CHAPTER 13

DEFINING *GINASTICA NATURAL* AND ITS INFLUENCES

With constant movement and varied connections between the movements, *Ginastica Natural* uses jiu-jitsu-based movements, breathing techniques, natural movements using the weight of the body itself and dynamic stretching and flexibility techniques.

ANIMAL MOVEMENTS

Animal movements are associated with different martial arts and after learning about some of these movements in Kempo classes, I conducted a biomechanical analysis on each one. Through this work, I was able to create a methodology to be applied during the classes. After that, I continued to use the names of the animals to identify the movements I developed for strength training. However, these represent a small part of the adult classes, since *Ginastica Natural* has hundreds of movements with specific names for each one.

In the program with classes for children, we work with a playful approach that includes games and stories, when we use animal movements more frequently. With *Ginastica*

Natural, we exercise the entire body, developing different physical qualities and psychomotor structures.

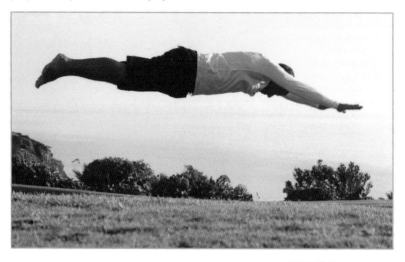

PROFESSOR ALVARO ROMANO IN GINASTICA NATURAL SUPERMAN PUSH UP

PSYCHOMOTOR STRUCTURES DEVELOPED THROUGH *GINASTICA NATURAL*

- Base Structures
- Handling / Locomotion and Muscle Tonus
- General Dynamics Coordination
- Ocular-Segment Coordination
- Balance
- Rhythm
- Structuring of Space-Time Organization in a Linear (movements in the same direction) and Structural Fashion (movements without any defined direction)
- Relaxation and Total Release from Actions

SOME PHYSICAL QUALITIES DEVELOPED DURING *GINASTICA NATURAL* CLASSES

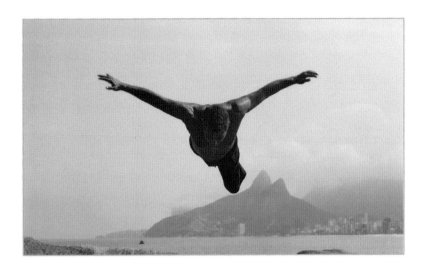

GINASTICA NATURAL FLY PUSH UP

- Dynamic Strength
- Static or Isometric Strength
- Explosive Strength
- Flexibility
- Stretching
- Speed
- Balance
- Coordination
- Rhythm
- Endurance
- Relaxation
- Efficiency

DEFINITIONS OF ALL TYPES OF STRENGTH DEVELOPED DURING *GINASTICA NATURAL* CLASSES

Dynamic Strength is a type of strength involving the force of the muscles in the moving limbs or strength in motion.

Static or Isometric Strength is strength explained through the production of heat, although without work in the form of movement.

Explosive Strength is the type of strength explained by the capacity to exercise a maximum amount of energy during an explosive act.

Flexibility is defined as the physical quality responsible for the range of movements available in a joint or group of joints.

Dynamic Flexibility is the physical quality expressed quickly by the maximum range of movement achieved by the motor muscles volitionally.

Static Stretching is that used generally during the initial phase of the class. It is the stretching that moves the muscle-joint group slowly, maintaining a posture with active muscle tension, determined by the greater range of voluntary movement, which makes use of the agonist muscle strength and antagonist muscle relaxation.

The Speed of the movement is an individual's maximum capacity to move from one point to another.

Static Balance is the type of balance achieved in a specific position.

Dynamic Balance is the type of balance achieved while in movement.

Recovered Balance is the physical quality that, in any position, explains the recovery of balance.

Coordination is the physical quality that represents the capacity to direct movement based on the conditions to resolve a diversified motor task.

Rhythm is the physical quality closely connected to the nervous system and present in all types of sports.

There are two types of Endurance, with prolonged and continuous duration, alternatively switching from an average to strong and weaker stimulus.

Differential Relaxation is the physical quality that allows for the relaxation of muscle groups that are not necessary when completing a specific motor task.

Agility is the skill to move the body in space. It is the skill of the entire body or a segment of the same to make a movement, changing directions quickly and precisely.

CHAPTER 14

QUALITY OF THE MOVEMENT AND BODY AWARENESS

To complete a movement effectively, we need to be fully concentrated on several aspects, such as correct breathing, and what leverage we can use to complete the movement perfectly. Consciously completing a sports-related movement or gesture tires us out less. An individual who goes for a simple jog, for example, may expend less energy when he or she understands that coordinating the arms with the legs helps drive the body forward better, that conscious breathing can relax the muscles of the face, similarly to a boxer who is in a certain position, whether one of dominance or in defense, or a surfer while catching a wave.

In different situations, body and breathing awareness can help us improve our performance. One good example would be during surfing competitions is the importance of rowing quickly with the arms and the surfer's intense movements to return to the site with waves. The surfer must use the correct breathing during this time, since this is crucial for recovering the effort made.

A jiu-jitsu fighter may save energy the same way when in a position of advantage or disadvantage. It is crucial to remain attentive to breathing and coordinate it with the completion of the movement. One important factor is that completing the movement slowly repeated times helps improve the range of the same with maximum concentration, and realizing that most times, a simple detail may lead to an improvement in this movement. Breathing while in motion helps us significantly improve our body awareness, but requires constant training. It is common to see people making a movement at a gym while talking or who look like they are lost in thought. Breathing while in motion helps improve the practice of the physical activity and can serve as a meditation in motion. The sensation of well-being will be much greater. I would like to cite examples like surfing and jiu-jitsu and the sensation they naturally provide, since when we practice these sports we are constantly focused on the activity and when this is the case, regardless of the exercise, we feel a big difference.

PRACTICING *GINASTICA NATURAL*

It is possible to practice *Ginastica Natural* at a range of different sites, either outdoors or indoors. No equipment or large spaces are required, depending on the number of people. Small, individual mats or the tatami can be used when larger areas are needed, for improved comfort and use by practitioners due to the movements on the ground, which represent the majority. I have given courses and classes in many places and under a range of different conditions, adapting the exercises. In my training, I have used all types of sites and floors/grounds. Due to the difficulties encountered in certain sites, I needed to train consciously, doing the exercises slowly and at a set speed. This was important training I did to improve and which offered me significant gains in terms of my body awareness.

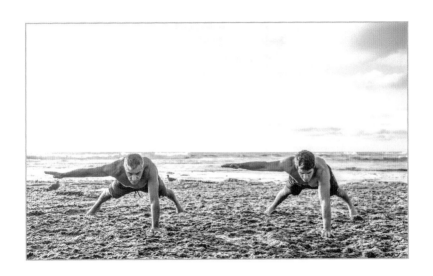

ONE HAND PUSH UP GINASTICA NATURAL EXERCISE

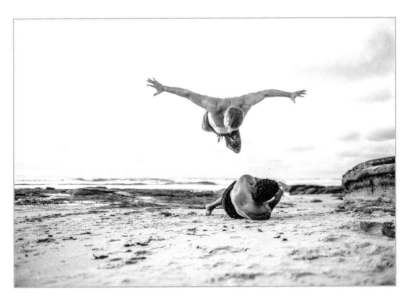

GINASTICA NATURAL PLYOMETRIC EXERCISE

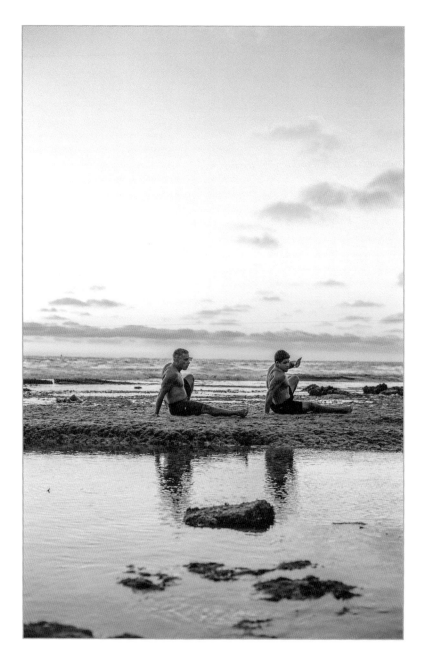

PROFESSORS ALVARO ROMANO AND RAPHAEL ROMANO

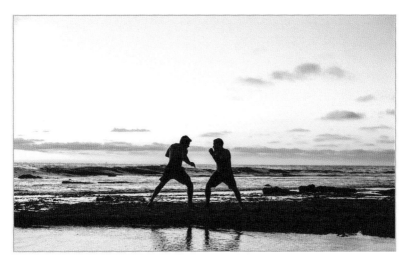

GINASTICA NATURAL FOR FIGHTERS EXERCISE

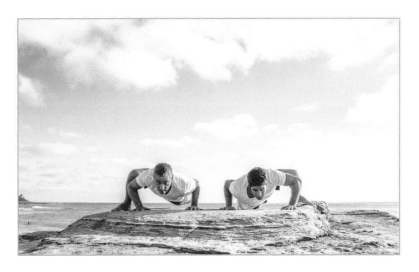

GINASTICA NATURAL SPIDER PUSH UP VARIATION

APPLYING *GINASTICA NATURAL* TO FITNESS, MMA AND SURFING

Ginastica Natural is functional training that uses the weight of the body itself and can be a different and effective option for use in all types of training programs.

It is ideal to diversify every activity, and this is what motivates students who are starting out or those who have practiced for longer periods. Most of the time, routine constitutes an obstacle for maintaining and attracting new students.

Seeking out different sites, varying the training and encouraging the student to practice activities that are not customary ones may have a very good result, since for some people, physical activity is an obligation.

Ginastica Natural is applied by many professors who are certified in functional exercise programs with equipment. The *Ginastica Natural* method of alternating traditional exercises with functional training equipment and with exercises that use the weight of the body has proven to be an innovative option in terms of breaking routine, with excellent results for building student loyalty.

However, there are some important factors for the professionals to evaluate, such as the student's goal – whether an athlete preparing for a competition or student looking to improve physical fitness, health and quality of life, the history, activities that he or she has practiced, and primarily, what he or she likes to do. There are students who have a past in sports, and resuming these activities can be a very good alternative for motivating them. It would be like an older person who trained in the martial arts or who surfed when younger and wants to resume this activity. However, they need to have the physical and mental conditions to do this. The training must evaluate the specific needs that must be developed to then begin, thereby prevent injuries or any other factors that could hinder the continued practice of the sport.

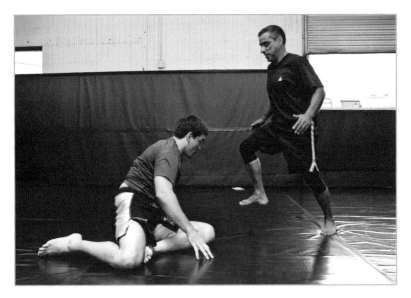

PROFESSOR ALVARO ROMANO TRAINING THE UFC FIGHTER DEMIAN MAIA IN SAN DIEGO, CA

CHAPTER 15

PROPOSALS FOR THE TRAINING PROGRAM

Research the preferred activity and try to do something in the beginning that is more pleasant for the student. Some enjoy working in the water while others do not. The idea is to adapt and gradually implement other training options. A satisfied and happy student, one who feels good due to his or her trust in the professor, is much more willing to accept suggestions. But for this to occur, we need to have diverse knowledge. If we limit ourselves to only one type of activity, there are but a few options. One example is the breathing techniques that few believe are important, but when students practice them, they see their value and are ultimately grateful.

Before any activity, people need to learn to breathe. These techniques help improve recovery and performance, and consequently, allow us to achieve our goals more quickly.

It is crucial to first practice these techniques to later teach them. This is because professionals from the area talk about their benefits, but do not know how to apply them.

Try and evaluate the training sites and check out the available options, such as the student's home, beaches, parks and even different gym options, to vary the activities and develop the programming.

CHAPTER 16

THE APPLICATION OF
GINASTICA NATURAL
DURING A TRAINING SESSION

Ginastica Natural techniques can be applied for all sports during different phases of a training session and can be the ideal warm-up, since we work several important physical qualities for this phase, primarily joint mobility. The ideal method would be a warm-up of around 30 minutes, including breathing techniques during this time, and a post-training recovery phase that lasts around 15 minutes, using specific exercises and release and relaxation techniques.

By the end of the warm-up session, the athlete should ideally be able to make any movement, both related to strength and wide range. It is common to see injuries occur at the start of a competition, when there can be an extreme situation and the athlete needs to make some of these movements but is not properly prepared for them.

There are cases of athletes only feeling warmed up a few minutes after the competition begins or after a few movements and this can weaken performance. The ideal thing for the athlete when he or she begins the competition is to already be at a higher level both physically and mentally when it comes to the warm-up. In this case, for any situation that may occur, his or her reaction will be without hesitation to use full potential.

Recovery is crucial during a training session. *Ginastica Natural* has several specific exercises that can be used in combination with breathing techniques. These are designed not only to recover the athlete, but also to ease any discomfort caused by the effort.

MOVEMENT AND SOME IMPORTANT ASPECTS TO CONSIDER BEFORE A COMPETITION

From a psychological aspect, it is important that this work be very well elaborated so that the athlete is most motivated at the right time, or in other words, the final minutes leading up to the competition. I try to explain to athletes by creating a comparison between this moment and the takeoff of a plane, which gradually warms up its turbines until reaching the point of maximum speed to be able to take off. For the athlete, as the moment of the competition grows closer, the adrenaline increases and this must be controlled. Therefore, at the right time, there can be that peak of motivation, concentration and focus. What is ideal is always peace of mind, the words to motivate must be well thought-out, since saying too much at the wrong time can have a negative effect. There are many of these situations in which athletes with great potential and very well-prepared lose competitions due to anxiety and stress. The days leading up to the competition are the most important. There are days on which emotions will make all the difference. Observing certain factors like the athlete's desire to be alone for a few moments, the time he or she wants to talk and the time required for privacy can help maintain that necessary peace of mind. That is why I think it is important for the athlete to always remain in a separate room at the sites reserved for the competition, and not have many people around all the time unless necessary. This often makes it harder for the athlete to rest. There are situations like a long-time friend watching the competition and wanting to be with the athlete the entire time, and the athlete feeling too embarrassed to say that he or she needs to rest. Real friends understand these needs, and that only the team is essential during that time. The fewer people around the athlete, the better. When the competition is about to begin, the whole strategy has to be ready. The encouraging words from the trainer must always be spoken calmly. Never incite anger, since this blinds the athlete and destroys his or her concentration. Feelings of anger cause the athlete to become completely "lost," forgetting all the strategy that has been developed and this can weaken his or her performance.

CHAPTER 17

SURFING AND *GINASTICA NATURAL*

Each day, more surfing athletes seek out *Ginastica Natural* as a training method, since with this training, they are not concerned about negatively affecting their performance by losing mobility and flexibility. These are crucial physical qualities for completing radical moves, and large waves and extreme situations make it necessary for these athletes to train all physical qualities. Using functional and weight training together with *Ginastica Natural* exercises are also an option that can help athletes boost their performance without losing flexibility.

Surfing is one of the sports that has most changed in terms of its physical training. Each day, athletes need to be better prepared and this is a factor that was not normally considered in the past. In order to be able to compete in all phases, athletes needed to be physically fit and focus on maintenance training during their long journeys around the world.

Training should also be focused on the preventive factor for injuries, since these are something increasingly common for athletes of this sport. During functional training, it is important to pay attention to certain details I have observed, such as reproducing the motions the athletes do for surf moves. This can overwork joints that are already very stressed and lead to a Repetitive Strain Injury (RSI). These athletes need to do precisely the opposite work, so as avoid stressing these joints, muscles and tendons. That is why flexibility and joint mobility training is crucial. Before and after every training session, it is important to always evaluate the athlete to discover any discomfort he or she is feeling, since we cannot run the risk of worsening an injury or even straining this joint. There are several functional training options in the pool that, depending on the situation, may be ideal since they offer no risks beyond being prophylactic.

It is important to remain attentive and focused on the ideal thing for each athlete: to finish the training with the desire to continue, with the sensation that they could have done more so they perform well the next day. Athletes who finish their training session exhausted, without the necessary recovery, may not rest sufficiently and will not do well during the following session, something that will only end up weakening their performance.

CHAPTER 18

GINASTICA NATURAL
AND PHYSICAL THERAPY

The relationship between my work and physical therapy began in 1985 after a serious injury to my knee during a jiu-jitsu competition in Rio de Janeiro. Of the many physicians I consulted, the majority recommended surgery. I scheduled an appointment with physical therapist Nilton Petrone, a professional who at the time was revolutionizing the way he treated patients. During this period, he saw patients at his home. After my first contact with him, I could already detect his knowledge and the innovations found in his treatment. I felt so very fortunate to be in contact with such a frontrunner of new methodology. I also knew that this would be a great learning experience.

This treatment was done without devices, and the equipment I did use was a simple bicycle tire chamber, flippers and a skateboard, which we used to work on strength, endurance and proprioception. Several different types of equipment were developed over the years that serve the same function, such as an exercise ball, elastic bands and others, but at the time these did not yet exist.

After approximately one month, I was cured and able to resume my activities. During this time, I brought him a black and white video, a very old one, which is available online to show him the work I was developing. It was a video with lots of movements on the floor; one I did myself for training and research of movements.

Surprised, he explained to me the importance of those exercises and how they could be used during rehabilitation. He went on to say that the way I presented them was innovative, and that they could be applied both during the patient's injury recovery phase as well as after recovery. The movements could be used before the individual resumed his or her activities, as if a transition between the two phases. This was important for starting to study a protocol of specific exercises to be applied during these treatment phases. From this moment on, *Ginastica Natural* underwent a major transformation, with new, diverse applications in different areas of human movement. We stayed in contact and a few years later, as Director of Physical Education and Physical Therapy Courses at Estácio de Sá University in Rio de Janeiro and head of the clinic located inside the university itself, he invited me to give classes for the Physical Therapy and Physical Education courses and take part in the recovery work for athletes by applying *Ginastica Natural*. This was done in his presence, together with a team of physical therapists.

I worked with many athletes and students, and all of them who needed it recovered through physical therapy integrated with *Ginastica Natural*.

Two important cases included MMA athlete Vitor Belfort in 1988, who recovered from a cervical spine injury, and famous soccer player Ronaldo "The Phenomenon," as he is known in

Brazil. We worked together to help the athlete recover from his knee surgery, allowing him to play during the World Soccer Cup in Asia in 2002. Brazil was champion and Ronaldo was the top scorer in the competition.

Due to the growing use of functional exercises in physical rehabilitation, *Ginastica Natural* has increasingly more representatives in physical therapy and its exercises are used in different cases for functional rehabilitation and special students.

CHAPTER 19

GINASTICA NATURAL EXERCISES

Now, we will conduct a kinesiological analysis on three exercises using frequently during *Ginastica Natural* classes.

The MONKEY movement adapted *to Ginastica Natural*

Starting Position

With a higher percentage of body mass over the lower limbs, support your hands on the ground.

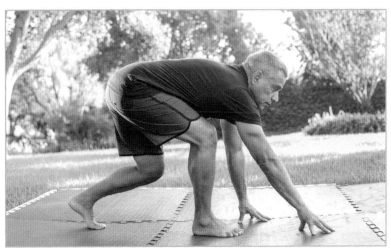

Movement

Legs flexed, moving the upper and lower limbs on the same time simultaneously, stretching the arms as far as possible

Analysis of the Movement

The Monkey Walk movement requires a series of kinesiological adaptations of our body to be done efficiently and correctly.

These adaptations allow us to gain strength using the anatomical curvature that is already in place, ensuring not only an improved motor skill experience when it comes to the large muscle masses, but also unique motor muscle contractions, such as for the lumbar paravertebral and semimembranosus gluteus muscles, biceps femoris and quadriceps.

Main joints involved in the movement:

- Hip – Flexing movement, with the femoral quadriceps as the agonist.
- Knee – Maintained in a semi-flexed position with use of anterior and posterior thigh muscles to stabilize the movement.
- Pelvic girdle – Maintained in retroversion during the initial position and anteversion during the movement itself.
- Backbone – The use of the paravertebral musculature area under strong tension, since the greater concentration of muscle mass in the lower limbs leads to the more intense use of this muscle group, primarily in the lower back region.

- Pectoral Girdle – action of the fixative muscles, since because it requires a load on the shoulders together with the movement of this joint, there is also the need for the proper development of the trapezius movements, scapular and rhomboids lifts in order to allow for this movement.

"Tiger Move" adapted for *Ginastica Natural*

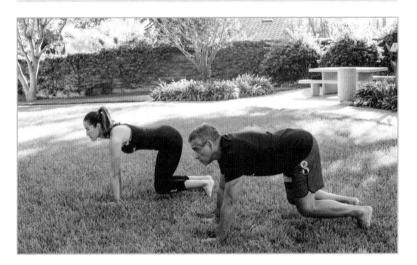

Starting Position

Leveling of the hips with the shoulders, supporting the hands and tips of the feet, equally distributing body weight

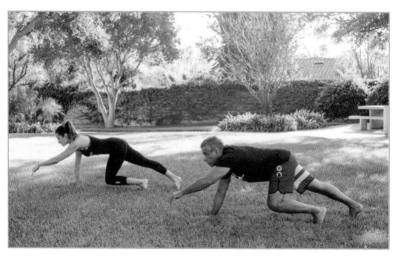

Movement

Step with one of the feet simultaneously with the arm on the same side, maintaining the hips level with the shoulders. Do not turn the pelvis.

Step with one of the feet simultaneously with the arm on the same side, maintaining the hips level with the shoulders. Do not turn the pelvis.

Analysis of the Movement

Due to the need to level out the pelvic girdle with the shoulders during the movement, the "Tiger" posture demands not only the excellent condition of the basic motor skill characteristics such as strength and endurance, but also kinesthetic perception. In other words, the person's ability to understand the movement and complete it correctly. The agonist or primary motor muscles used in the movement, as well as the stabilizers, play an important role in terms of distributing body mass and positioning the center of gravity.

Study of the main joints involved in the movement:

Pelvic Girdle, Hips, Knees, Pectoral Girdle, Shoulders and Elbows

Main Movements:

- Hips – flexion and extension movement
- Knee – flexion and extension
- Shoulders – flexion and extension
- Elbows – flexion and extension

Main Muscles:

- Hips, iliac, sartorius, rectus femoris, pectíneus, biceps femoris, semitendinosus, semimembranosus, rectus femoris, vastus intermedius, vastus medialis, deltoid, pectoralis major and minor, biceps and triceps.
- The rectus abdominis and paravertebral are muscle groups that have a stabilizing function

"Horse Kick" movement adapted for *Ginastica Natural*

You can clearly see that it is a movement that requires a very advanced motor skill experience, since there is an inversion associated with the support over the ground. This requires the practitioner to have a better perception of the reflexes required to stand the body up to achieve the desired performance, although without compromising his or her safety.

Starting Position:

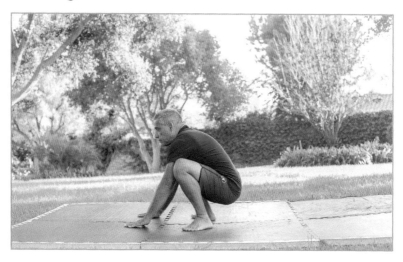

Four (4) limbs supported on the ground, with the body in a crouching position and with the highest percentage of body mass over the low limbs, aiming to use a maximum range so as to balance the body's center of gravity.

Movement:

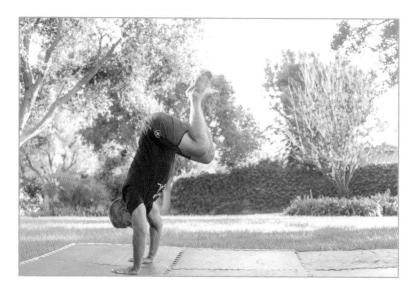

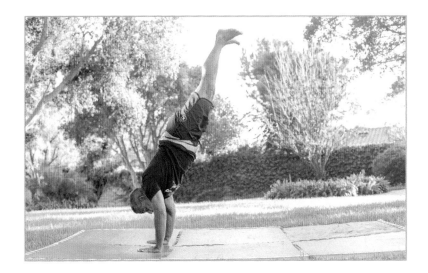

When starting the movement, there is a slight tilt of the torso frontward, which causes the center of gravity to leave its support base. This leads to a state of unbalance, while at the same time, we also have a vigorous contracting of the paravertebral and gluteal muscles, popliteus muscles and femoral quadriceps so that we can transfer the body weight to the upper balanced limbs and project the lower limbs and torso upward.

- Return to the starting position while maintaining your balance.

- Main joints involved in the movement:

- Shoulder–Eccentric contraction of the shoulder joint extensor muscles. Allows for the stabilization of the body.

- Elbow–Triceps and biceps brachii, which contract for the fixation of this joint.

- Pectoral Girdle-The muscles responsible for fixating the pectoral girdle contract, but we believe there is a significant demand of the trapezium and rhomboid for the scapular adduction.

- Backbone-Extension by contracting the paravertebral and gluteus muscles.

- Hips-The hips are extended upward by contracting the gluteus maximus, biceps femoris, semitendinosus and semimembranosus.

- Knee-The knee is extended by contracting the femoral quadriceps.

GINASTICA NATURAL BAR TRAINING

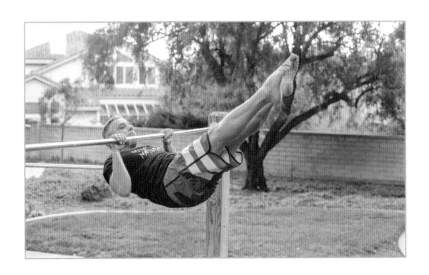

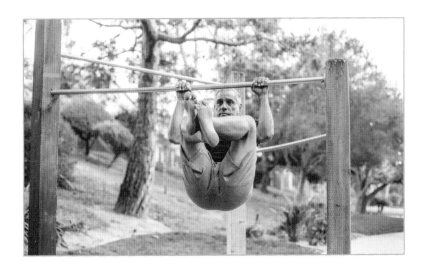

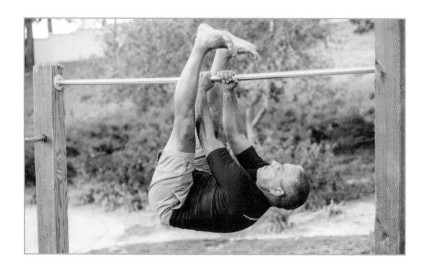

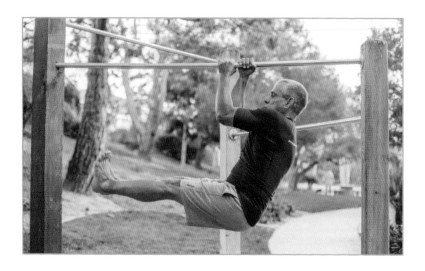

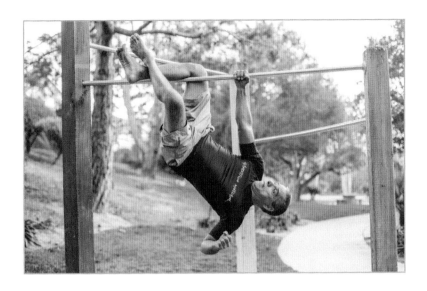

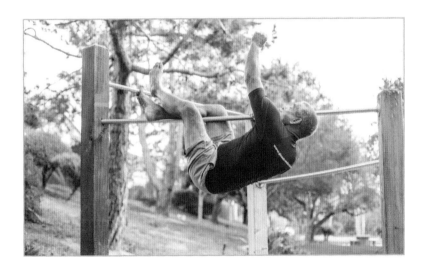

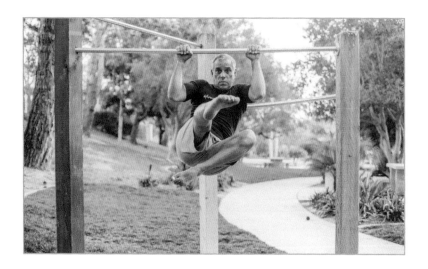

BIBLIOGRAPHY

Gomes Tubino Manuel Jose, *Metodologia Científica do Treinamento desportivo* (editora Inbrasa, Brazil, 1980)

Hermógenes, Jose, *Auto Perfeição com Hatha Yoga* (Editora, Freitas Bastos, Brazil, 1963)

Dantas, Estelio HM, *Pisicofisiologia*, Shape 2009

Printed in Great Britain
by Amazon

57528196R00091